Healthy Living

Paleo Diet
for Beginners

21-Day Meal Plan
105 Quick & Easy Recipes
Tips for Success

Madison Miller

ISBN: 9781790164295

Printed in the United States

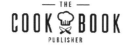

CONTENTS

INTRODUCTION

Over the past year, my family and I have changed our typical North American way of eating to follow the paleo diet revolution. This basically means that we eat the food our hunter-gatherer ancestors from the Paleolithic Era did while adapting it to the modern times we live in. We focus on foods such as tree-ripened fresh fruits, fresh veggies, grass-fed animal meats, wild fish, nuts, seeds, and plant roots. If our ancestors could hunt them or gather them, they are included. Therefore, we have eliminated all processed and refined foods, grains, and legumes from our diet. We use lots of spices and herbs for flavors and healthy fats such as avocados and olive oil to make delicious meals the whole family enjoy.

We also opted for more organic produce, meat, and fish. Although it may be more expensive, it is definitively a healthier choice. Pesticides, antibiotics, hormones, and non-organic fertilizers and chemicals are not used in the production process. The whole idea behind the paleo diet is to eat healthily and, consequently, feel better. It should be said that the paleo diet is not about eating tons of meat and fat, but rather, adopting healthy eating habits and balancing your consumption of food between lean proteins found in fish, meats and seafood, healthy fats, vegetables, and fruits.

We noticed that it took us a good two weeks to get used to our new diet. It definitively takes more time and energy to follow a paleo lifestyle, considering the amount of time needed for cooking, food preparation, and grocery shopping. It also is more costly if you buy only organic fruits and vegetables, grass-fed meats, and wild fish and seafood. However, the health benefits are definitely worth it.

Benefits of the Paleo Diet

Before we started on our paleo lifestyle journey, both my husband and I were overweight and out of shape with very low energy levels. We would typically go to work, eat, crash in front of the television, and fall asleep...and start over again the next day. The paleo diet has changed this for us.

Here is a short list of advantages we have noticed regarding health since switching to the paleo diet.

Losing weight and maintaining an ideal weight level

Healthy weight loss is considered to be the most sought-after benefit achieved from following a paleo diet. The concept behind this is quite simple. By eating fewer carbohydrates and eliminating refined sugars, unhealthy fats, and processed and excessively salty foods from our diet, we prevent ourselves from overeating. This causes the sugar cravings to stop, and our insulin level normalizes, making our body more likely to break down fats instead of storing them. Your metabolism improves, and because your intake is healthier and rich in nutrients, you feel full faster and eat less. The diet also makes it easy to maintain your ideal weight as you are fuelling your body with real and nourishing foods.

Promotes good digestion

The fiber-rich paleo diet greatly improves the health of your digestive system. Since you have eliminated from your diet all grains and legumes, the main irritants to a healthy intestinal flora, your digestive system will thank you. You feel lighter and less bloated.

Boosts and regulates energy level

Following the paleo diet makes you feel more energetic. As a matter of fact, this is the diet that provided our ancestors with the unlimited energy to walk miles and miles each day, hunting predators and lifting heavy weights.

This is the most important benefit for me. I have tons of energy to start and finish any project I think about, like writing this book. It was like a lethargic brain fog was lifted as the weeks passed. I feel energized, and I sleep better.

Similarly, we noticed that our mood swings were more even throughout the day. We did not feel the ups and downs we did before. No more sugar fixes at four o'clock or little pick-me-ups in late mornings. It's a great feeling.

Reduces the risk of chronic diseases

Just by stopping ingesting processed and refined foods, and the huge amount of sugars and salt that goes with them, you will boost your body's resistance to diseases such as heart disease, diabetes, and even cancer.

In his book, *The Paleo Diet*, Dr. Loren Cardain, one of the leading experts on Paleolithic nutrition, has concluded that our hunter-gatherer ancestors did not suffer from the same chronic sicknesses that our modern society faces now. He explains: *"The nutritional qualities of modern processed foods and foods introduced during the Neolithic period are discordant with our ancient and conservative genome. This genetic discordance ultimately manifests itself as various chronic illnesses, which have been dubbed "diseases of civilization." By severely reducing or eliminating these foods and replacing them with a more healthful cuisine, possessing nutrient qualities more in line with the foods our ancestors consumed, it is possible to improve health and reduce the risk of chronic disease."*

We highly recommend reading Cardain's book as it clearly explains the basis for the paleo diet.

Several studies have shown that a paleo diet helps reduce high blood pressure and cholesterol levels. My husband's high blood pressure is now under control, and all he did was change his eating habits.

Reduces inflammation

The healthy food choices of the paleo diet have been proven to reduce inflammation in the body, particularly of the joints and the pain associated with it in diseases such as arthritis. This is definitely an advantage I noticed only after a few weeks. The morning stiffness I usually felt started to decrease significantly.

There are many more advantages to following a paleo diet and lifestyle. I have compiled only a few here, those that we noticed the most, to show how amazing you can feel when you follow this way of nourishment. I encourage anyone to further research this topic.

EATING THE PALEO WAY

We have put together a 21-day recipe cookbook that includes 21 breakfasts, 21 snacks, 21 lunches, 21 dinners, and 21 desserts to help anyone get started on their paleo diet journey. Yes, dessert! It's still something I find hard to let go of, but when you use ingredients that nourish you, there is nothing wrong with having some sweets!

Like with any change in your nutrition plan, it is imperative that you check with your doctor first to see if this diet can suit you.

What to Eat

An ideal paleo diet plate could look like this: more than half for vegetables, a quarter for lean proteins, and the remaining separated between healthy fats and fruits.

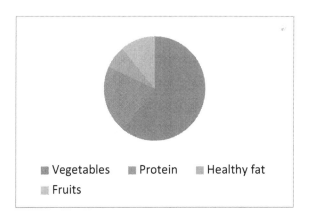

When you start following a nutrition plan based on the paleo diet, you must be aware of the food that you should be eating, the food to avoid, and the food to eat in moderation. The 21-day eating plan presented in this book hinges on these three food lists.

There are a lot of gray areas about which foods are acceptable or not in a paleo diet. One such area is starchy vegetables such as the sweet potato. We include this vegetable on the list of green foods because it is rich in nutrients and vitamins. I think you have to use your common sense here and judge for yourself what you are ready to accept or not in your own paleo diet. We also indulge in dark chocolate that has 70 percent cacao or more, as it is recognized as a good source of antioxidants. We also drink teas, herbal teas, and coffee (without the dairy added, though). Also, we use organic maple syrup and raw honey as natural sweeteners. We do not drink alcohol at all, but you could consider it with dry wines and non-grain-based spirits. The debate is still open.

Healthy Carbohydrates, Proteins, Fats, Condiments

Carbohydrates – Vegetables

Artichoke, asparagus, beet, broccoli, Brussels sprout, cabbage (all varieties), carrots, cauliflower, celery, chard, collards greens, cucumber, eggplant, endive, fennel, herbs (all varieties), kale, leek, lettuce, mushroom, onions, parsnip, peppers (all varieties), pumpkin, okra, radish, rutabaga, shallot, spinach, squash (all varieties), sweet potato, tomatillo, tomato, turnip.

Carbohydrates – Fruits

Apple, apricot, banana, berries (acai, blueberry, blackberry, boysenberry, cranberry, elderberry, gooseberry, huckleberry, mulberry, raspberry),clementine, currant, cherry, damson, feijoa, grape, grapefruit, guava, Jamul, kiwi, kumquat, lemon, lime, lychee, mango, melon (all varieties), nectarine, orange, papaya, passion fruit, peach, pear, persimmon, plum, pineapple, pomegranate, pomelo, redcurrant, star fruit, watermelon.

Proteins (unprocessed, preferably grass fed lean cuts, organic, free range...)

Beef,
Fish – any kind, preferably wild fish
Eggs (all varieties)
Lamb
Pork
Poultry – chicken, duck, quail, pigeon, turkey
Seafood – clams, crab, crawfish, crayfish, lobster, mussels, oysters, scallops, shrimp
Organ meat – liver, marrow, sweetbreads, tongue
Veal
Wild game meat – all varieties such as bison, buffalo, rabbit, venison, elk, emu, boar...

Fats

Avocado, avocado oil
Flaxseed oil
Ghee (clarified butter)
Nuts - almond, Brazilian, cashews, chestnut, coconut, hazelnut, macadamia, pecans, pine nuts, pistachios, walnut
Nuts - oils and butters - almonds, cashews, coconut, hazelnut, macadamia, pistachios, walnut
Olive, olive oil extra virgin & cold pressed
Seeds – seed oils - flaxseed, grape, pumpkin, sesame, sunflower

Condiments

All natural mustards, coconut amino, vinegar, all spices and herbs, sea salt in moderation, coconut milk (unsweetened), and almond milk (unsweetened).

Food to Eat in Moderation

Dried fruits (because of their high sugar content) – 2 oz per day Raw honey, organic maple syrup

Healthy fats

Nuts – taking into account the high-fat content of nuts, it is easy to go overboard; we recommend 1 serving per day, about 4 oz.

Dark chocolate – with high content of pure cocoa 70 percent or above, in moderation

Proteins

Fattier cuts of any meats

Food to Avoid

If it comes in a package, you probably should not eat it because it has been processed. These products usually contain unhealthy sugars, fats, too much salt, gluten, grains, and preserving agents. Read the ingredients list carefully.

All dairy foods – butter, cheese, milk, powdered milk, yogurt, cream, cream cheese, ice cream

All cereal grains – wheat, corn, barley, oats, maize, millet, rice, rye, sorghum, quinoa, buckwheat, amaranth, wild rice

All refined processed foods – cookies, pastries, breakfast cereals, candy, sodas, energy drinks, ketchup, processed meat and deli, chips, fries, pickled foods

High-glycemic starchy vegetables – Potatoes, tapioca, manioc

All legumes – all beans (adzuki, black, black-eyed, fava, butter, calico, cannellini, garbanzo (chickpeas), kidney, lima, mung, navy, pinto, soy, white); all peas (sugar snap peas, peas, snow peas, green beans, split peas); lentils, peanuts

All soybean products – tofu, edamame, miso, tempeh, soya sauce, etc.

Processed fats – corn oil, peanut oil, canola oil, store-bought mayonnaise

What to Drink on the Paleo Diet

Getting enough hydration is very important in any diet.
Water – most of your hydration should come from water, preferably filtered water

Other choices include:
Coconut water – natural and unprocessed
Juices from fresh fruits and fresh vegetables
Herbal teas, coffee

Freshly squeezed fruit juices should be consumed in moderation because of their high content of natural sugar, which can offset your blood sugar level and insulin production.

ORGANIZING YOUR PANTRY AND KITCHEN

Organizing your pantry and your kitchen will be essential to being successful when you start your paleo journey. This helps because it will stop you from being tempted by a particular prohibited food item and encourage you to eat the healthy alternatives.

In order to implement a paleo diet in your household, you will need to organize your kitchen first. For that, you should take out all the items that are on the to-be-avoided list. This involves taking out all the dairy products along with sugar, grains (wheat, buckwheat, legumes, corn, rice, beans), inorganic foods and artificial foods (like soy sauces, ketchup, store-bought dressings, Worcestershire sauce). You can then start building a paleo-friendly kitchen. First, make sure you stock up on the dry ingredients you will need frequently. I would start with olive oil (extra virgin and cold pressed), coconut oil, coconut butter, avocado oil, flaxseed oil (to keep refrigerated), some of your favourite raw nuts and seeds, coconut flour, almond meal, almond flour, coconut milk (unsweetened), almond milk (unsweetened), almond butter, cashew butter, mustards, coconut amino (can be used to replace the salty soya sauce), vinegar, spices, raw honey, organic maple syrup and sea salt. For refrigerated produce and meat, I would only get those as you plan your meals. Eat them as fresh as possible.

If you are the only one in your household following a paleo diet, it makes it more difficult, but certainly not impossible. You will have to reserve some space in your pantry and your fridge to store the healthy foods you will be eating. When your household members find out how great you feel and look, they'll want to join you on this journey!

TIPS TO MAKE IT EASIER

Planning what you will eat a few days in advance is the key to staying on top of your paleo diet. If you know what you are making and the time it will take you, it is much easier to make your time fit your schedule. I always plan a week at a time. It allows me to see how much time is needed every day for meal preparation, cooking time, grocery shopping.

Double up on recipes that can easily be frozen such as stews, casseroles, and soups. When you don't feel like cooking, you know you have something ready to use. It will happen, so be prepared!

If I know I have to use chopped vegetables, I typically do all my chopping after I have planned my week and done all the shopping. I like to do this with namely, onions, garlic, ginger, and vegetables. You can easily freeze chopped vegetables, preferably by portions used per meal.

It is also useful to have some pre-cooked meat, poultry, or fish on hand to make quick lunches or for quick bites on the go. I will typically roast a chicken with my favorite seasoning on the weekend, and use it for salad, wraps, and even breakfast protein.

If I go to a farm to buy my grass-fed meats, I'll freeze by the portion in a zip-lock bag, and then mark the date and the kind of meat.

At the grocery store, if I know what I am eating for that week, I will only buy what's on my list. This keeps me from buying too much and having food go to waste. It is also a good idea to visit your local farmer's market in season. Buy local. Most grocery stores now have a section for organic ingredients or go to your local organic food store like Whole Food.

You can still eat out on the paleo diet, although it can be challenging. Ask questions about the ingredients used in preparing dishes you want to order to make sure they conform to your healthy eating habits. Ask your waiter not to bring any bread. Skip the potato or starches that usually comes when ordering meat or fish and seafood dishes. If ordering a salad, ask for olive oil and vinegar on the side for the dressing. Order your protein grilled with no sauce and avoid all dishes containing cheese or dairy products. Avoid all deep-fried dishes or any breaded ingredients. Ask for your vegetables to be steamed.

21 DAYS PALEO EATING PLAN

The meal plan that follows is a suggestion for having a well-assorted menu all week long. You can click on any meal from this plan to go directly to the recipe page.

21 Days to Make It into a Habit

Remember that this diet is not a magic wand that will transform your life all of a sudden. You have to be consistent and stick to the diet for a period of time before you can feel and see differences. This is a change in your lifestyle to improve your health and to know and control what goes into your body. As you notice the improvements to your health and the way you look and feel; you'll want to commit to the paleo lifestyle. There will be a period of adjustment as your body adjusts to your new diet. As we are not health professionals, we can only share our experience. As we started to eat more fiber with plenty of fresh vegetables and fruits than we ever had before, our intestinal tracts reacted in the first two weeks with frequent visits to the bathroom!

You may feel uncomfortable, experience some headaches, and just feel cranky because you want your sugar fix. However, this will pass, and then you'll feel great, and full of energy.

There is a saying that it takes you 21 days to change a behavior into a new one. If you eat paleo for 21 days, it will become a habit. By putting all the odds of success on your side, like organizing your kitchen, getting rid of temptations, planning your meals in advance, and thinking positively about how your health is improving every day, it will tilt the balance in your favor. Visualize yourself healthy, lighter, feeling and looking your best ever.

The 21-Days Meal Plan

B= Breakfast; S= Snack; L=Lunch; D= Dinner; De= Dessert

Week 1

Monday:
- **B=** Vegetable Frittata; **(p27)**
- **S:** Fresh Berry Cereal; **(p84)**
- **L:** Salmon, Spinach & Apple Salad; **(p93)**
- **D:** Piri Piri Chicken ; **(p129)**
- **De:** Quick Chocolate Bonbon **(p177)**

Tuesday
- **B=** Grainless Blueberry Waffles; **(p29)**
- **S:** Blueberry & Spinach Smoothie; **(p90)**
- **L:** Sautéed Coconut Chicken; **(p95)**
- **D:** Nutty Tilapia Fillets; **(p131)**
- **De:** Cherry and Almond Butter Milkshake **(p181)**

Wednesday
- **B=** Pink & Delicious Pancakes ; **(p31)**
- **S:** Pumpkin Pie Spice with Sweet Potato; **(p91)**
- **L:** Macadamia Hummus with Vegetables; **(p101)**
- **D:** Roasted Beef with Nutty Vegetables; **(p139)**
- **De:** Ginger Brownies **(p179)**

Thursday
- **B=** Scramble Eggs à la Provençale ; **(p33)**
- **S:** Banana Chips; **(p85)**
- **L:** The Big Salad; **(p97)**
- **D:** Tandoori Chicken Drumsticks & Mango Chutney **(p133)**
- **De:** Maple Paleo Bread **(p201)**

Friday
  B: Crustless Mini Bacon Quiches; **(p57)**
  S: Fruity Cinnamon Smoothie; **(p86)**
  L: Mushroom Cream Soup; **(p117)**
  D: Roasted Salmon with Bacon; **(p167)**
  De: Creamy Berries **(p203)**

Saturday
  B: Pumpkin Breakfast Pancakes; **(p59)**
  S: Spicy Fruit Salad **(p82)**
  L: Brussels Sprouts & Bacon with Tandoori Drumsticks; **(p110)**
  D: Pork chops with Apples; **(p151)**
  De: Carrot Cake Bites **(p204)**

Sunday
  B= Popeye Breakfast Pie; **(p41)**
  S: Fresh fruits with Mint & Lime; **(p89)**
  L: Grilled Shrimps Salad **(p107)**
  D: Honey Mustard Beef; **(p175)**
  De: Crunchy Baked Apples **(p195)**

Week 2
Monday:
  B: Apple Sauce Seasoned Paleo Pancakes; **(p35)**
  S: Spicy Nuts; **(p73)**
  L: Carrot Soup; **(p103)**
  D: Stuffed Sea Bass; **(p135)**
  De: Banana with Coconut & Almond Butter **(p182)**
Tuesday
  B: Cocoa Almond Squares; **(p47)**
  S: Green Smoothie; **(p75)**
  L: Grilled Chicken with Olive and Tomato Topping; **(p105)**
  D: Baked Beef with Vegetables; **(p147)**
  De: Paleo Pumpkin Muffins **(p183)**

15

Wednesday

   B: Little Black Dress Omelet; **(p39)**

   S: Tropical Delight Fruit Bowl; **(p76)**

   L: *Sautéed Leeks with Salmon;* **(p123)**

   D: Paleo Orange Chicken; **(p143)**

   De: Creamy Banana Treat with Cranberries and Coconut milk **(p186)**

Thursday

   B: Paleo Classic Apple & Spice Muffins; (p37)

   S: Seasoned Seaweeds; (p77)

   L: Cucumber & Watermelon Salad; (p115)

   D: Ground Beef with Kale; (p152)

   De: Berries with Almonds (p187)

Friday

   B: You Could Eat Some All Day Pancakes **(p43)**

   S: Apple Chips; **(p79)**

   L: Delightful Vegetable Medley Soup; **(p111)**

   D: Tilapia with Thai Curry; **(p141)**

   De: Coconut Whipped Cream **(p185)**

Saturday

   B: Mammoth Breakfast Casserole; **(p45)**

   S: Spicy Cauliflower; **(p81)**

   L: Salmon & Asparagus Salad, **(p115)**

   D: Beef Goulash; **(p145)**

   De: Sweet & Salty Chocolate Barks **(p188)**

Sunday

   B: Caveman Breakfast Hash; **(p50)**

   S: Carrot Smoothie; **(p80)**

   L: Paleo Prawns with Tomato Sauce; **(p113)**

   D: Herb-Crusted Pork Tenderloin; **(p149)**

   De: Honey Coated Walnuts & peaches **(p189)**

Week 3
Monday:
 B: Glorious Morning Smoothie; **(p49)**
 S: *Healthy Granola Bars*; **(p69)**
 L: Chicken, Tomato, Mint & Basil salad; **(p120)**
 D: Butterfish with Lemongrass; **(p161)**
 De: Apple Pudding with Coconut Whipped Cream **(p191)**

Tuesday
 B: Poblano Pepper Omelet; **(p61)**
 S: Watermelon & Kiwi with Fresh Herbs; **(p74)**
 L: Paleo Tuna Salad; **(p119)**
 D: Sautéed Juicy Pork Tenderloin with Peaches; **(p157)**
 De: Raspberry Ice Cream **(p193)**

Wednesday
 B: Breakfast Paleo Waffles; **(p53)**
 S: Kale Chips; **(p83)**
 L: Broccoli & Pine Nuts Soup; **(p109)**
 D: Baked Chicken with Olives; **(p162)**
 De: Almond Florentine **(p190)**

Thursday
 B: Jalapeño Scrambled Eggs with Cherry Tomatoes; **(p63)**
 S: S & B Smoothie; **(p78)**
 L: Chicken & Spinach; **(p125)**
 D: Liver with Onions; **(p165)**
 De: Chocolate Pudding **(p194)**

Friday
  B: Peachy Pancakes; **(p65)**
  S: Primal Trail Mix; **(p87)**
  L: Quick and Easy Egg Salad Wrap **(p121)**
  D: Fish Curry with Bananas **(p173)**
  De: Banana Bites **(p200)**

Saturday
  B: Hungry Man Steak & Bacon Hash; **(p55)**
  S: St-Patrick Day Smoothie; **(p88)**
  L: Lemon Grilled Chicken; **(p127)**
  D: Hearty Beef and Vegetable Stew; **(p159)**
  De: Coconut Squares **(p197)**

Sunday
  B: Mexican Scramble; **(p67)**
  S: Paleo Beef Jerky; **(p71)**
  L: Simple Salmon Salad **(p126)**
  D: Primal Chicken Fajitas; **(p163)**
  De: Baked Pears **(p199)**

BREAKFAST RECIPES

Vegetable Frittata

Serves: 4
Prep Time: 15 minutes
Cooking Time: 20 minutes

Ingredients
4 eggs
30 ml (2 tablespoons) olive oil
1 onion, chopped
1 garlic clove, minced
125 ml (½ cup) carrots, thinly sliced
125 ml (½ cup) red bell pepper, deseeded, julienne
1 zucchini, thinly sliced
125 ml (½ cup) baby spinach, chopped
15 ml (1 tablespoon) fresh basil, chopped
Sea salt and freshly ground pepper to taste
Fresh parsley, chopped for sprinkle

Directions:
1. In a bowl, whisk the eggs vigorously until fluffy, about 2 minutes.
2. Heat oil in a frying non-stick pan, sauté onions and garlic for 2-3 minutes on high heat until tender.
3. Lower the heat to medium. Add red bell peppers, zucchini, spinach, and tomatoes. Cook for 5 minutes until vegetables are crisply tender. Add eggs and basil. Season with salt and pepper to taste. Cook for 10-15 minutes on medium low heat until the eggs are done.
4. Cut into wedges, sprinkle with parsley, and serve hot.

Nutritional Information (per serving)
Calories: 258
Fat total: 22.1g, saturated fat: 6.5g
Carbohydrates: 8.0g, dietary fiber: 2.6g
Sugars: 3.8g, protein: 7.2g

Primal Blueberry Waffles

Serves: 4
Prep Time: 15 minutes
Cooking Time: 12-15 minutes

Ingredients:
250 ml (1 cup) blueberries
3 eggs, separated
250 ml (1 cup) almond flour
60 ml (¼ cup) almond milk
1 teaspoon vanilla extract
30 ml (2 tablespoons) olive oil
Maple syrup to sprinkle (optional – can be replaced by raw honey)

Directions:
1. Grease the waffle maker with olive oil or coconut butter, and pre-heat it.
2. In a mixing bowl, using a hand electric beater, whisk the egg whites on high speed until they form stiff peaks, about 2-3 minutes.
3. In another bowl, combine the egg yolks, the almond milk, and vanilla extract. Add the coconut flour and salt and olive oil. Mix well until you have a smooth batter.

4. Incorporate 1/3 of the egg whites into the batter, mixing well. Add another 1/3 of the egg whites, and fold it in the batter until they are well incorporated. Repeat. You should have a light and fluffy batter.
5. Pour about 1/2 cup of the batter into the waffle maker, close the lid, and let it cook according to the manufacturer instructions.
6. To serve, top each waffle with blueberries, and drizzle with maple syrup or raw honey.

Nutritional Information (per serving)
Calories: 448
Fat total: 37.4g, saturated fat: 21.5g
Carbohydrates: 24.3g, dietary fiber: 6.3g
Sugars: 13.9g, protein: 9.2g

Pink & Delicious Pancakes

Serves: 4
Prep Time: 10 minutes
Cooking Time: 10 minutes

Ingredients:
250 ml (1 cup) fresh raspberries
4 eggs
250 ml (1 cup) almond meal
125 ml (½ cup) unsweetened almond milk
1 teaspoon vanilla extract
10 ml (2 teaspoons) baking powder
2.5 ml (½ teaspoon) ground cinnamon
30 ml (2 tablespoons) coconut oil
30 ml (2 tablespoons) olive oil

Maple syrup for drizzle or fresh fruits with raw honey for garnish

Directions:
1. In a bowl, whisk together the raspberries and the eggs.
2. Mix in almond milk, olive oil, and vanilla extract
3. In another bowl, whisk together almond meal, baking powder, and cinnamon.
4. Gradually add the dry ingredients with the egg and blueberries. Combine well using a whisk.
5. Melt the coconut butter in a medium-sized frying pan on high heat. Spoon about 30 ml (2 tablespoons) of the batter into the pan. Cook for 2-3 minutes or until slightly golden on each side.
6. Drizzle with maple syrup or fresh fruits with raw honey for garnish and serve.

Nutritional Information (per serving)
Calories: 448
Fat total: 37.4g, saturated fat: 21.5g
Carbohydrates: 24.3g, dietary fiber: 6.3g
Sugars: 13.9g, protein: 9.2g

Scramble Eggs à la Provençale

Serves: 4
Prep Time: 5 minutes
Cooking Time: 10 minutes

Ingredients:
125 ml (½ cup) onions, chopped
125 ml (½ cup) tomatoes, chopped
4 eggs
125 ml (½ cup) fresh basil leaves, chopped
2.5 ml (½ teaspoon) dried Provençale herb mix
Sea salt and freshly ground pepper to taste
30 ml (2 tablespoons) coconut oil

Directions
1. In a mixing bowl, whisk the eggs until fluffy. Add Provençale herbs.
2. Melt the coconut oil in a medium frying pan, Add onions, and sauté for 2-3 minutes until the onions are fragrant and tender. Add tomatoes and basil leaves. Season with salt and pepper.
3. Add eggs to the pan, and cook for 3-5 minutes until the eggs are not runny anymore, stirring occasionally to scramble the eggs.
4. Serve hot with paleo-approved breakfast sausages or bacon strips, if desired.

Nutritional Information (per serving – no bacon or sausage)
Calories: 251
Fat total: 22.4g, saturated fat: 14.5g
Carbohydrates: 2.2g, dietary fiber: 0.5g
Sugars: 1.7g, protein: 11.5g

Applesauce Seasoned Paleo Pancakes

Serves: 2
Prep Time: 10 minutes
Cooking Time: 10 minutes

Ingredients
250 ml (1 cup) unsweetened applesauce, preferably homemade or organic
250 ml (1 cup) almond meal
3 eggs
60 ml (¼ cup) almond milk
2.5 ml (½ teaspoon) baking powder
5 ml (1 teaspoon) vanilla extract
1 ml (¼ teaspoon) ground nutmeg
1 ml (¼ teaspoon) ground cinnamon
30 ml (2 tablespoons) melted coconut oil
Olive oil for frying

Directions:
1. Beat eggs and applesauce together in a mixing bowl. Add vanilla, almond milk, olive oil.
2. Mix almond milk and vanilla extract with egg and potatoes.
3. In another bowl, mix together almond meal, baking powder, ground nutmeg, and ground cinnamon.
4. Gradually add the dry ingredients to the eggs mixture, and combine well.
5. Heat about 1 tablespoon of olive oil in a medium frying non-stick pan. When the oil is hot, spoon about 60 ml (1/4 cup) of this batter into the pan, and cook for 2-3 minutes on each side until slightly golden.
6. Serve the pancakes hot with a drizzle of organic maple syrup or fresh fruits with raw honey.

Nutritional Information (per serving)
Calories: 407
Fat total: 31.7g, saturated fat: 7.7g,
Carbohydrates: 22.5g, dietary fiber: 7.9g
Sugars: 2.9g, protein: 13.8g

Paleo Classic Apple and Spice Muffins

Prep time: 15 minutes
Cooking time:
Yields 12 muffins

Ingredients:
2 cups almond flour
2 teaspoons baking powder
3 apples, peeled and shredded
2 tablespoons maple syrup
¾ cup coconut milk
2 large eggs
2 tablespoons coconut oil
1 teaspoon cinnamon
1/8 teaspoon nutmeg
Vegetable cooking spray

Directions:
1. Preheat your oven to 180°C/350°F. Grease muffin tin with cooking spray.
2. In a bowl, mix dry ingredients together well.
3. In another bowl, mix all wet ingredients, until well combined. Add the mixture to the dry ingredients and whisk well.

4. Add the minced apple to the batter and mix well. Pour the batter into each the muffin hole until they are 3/4 full.
5. Bake for around 18-20 minutes, until cooked thoroughly. You can check by inserting a toothpick in the middle of one of the muffin.

Nutrition Information per muffin:
Calories: 168
Carbs: 17 g; Fat: 5.5 g
Protein: 3 g, Sugars: 16.3g

Little Black Dress Omelet

Serves: 4
Prep Time: 10 minutes
Cooking Time: 10 minutes

Ingredients:
250 ml (1 cup) onion
250 ml (1 cup) spinach
1 tomato, sliced
30 ml (2 tablespoons) coconut oil
8 egg whites
Sea salt and freshly ground pepper to taste
Tomato and cucumber slices for garnish

Directions:
1. Heat the oil in a large skillet, Cook onions for 2-3 minutes until fragrant and tender. Add the tomatoes and spinach, and sauté for another 2-3 minutes.
2. Add egg whites to the vegetables. Season with salt and pepper to taste. Cook for 2-3 minutes until the sides

become golden brown, and the omelet is fully cooked. Fold half the omelet on the other side.
3. Serve with tomato and cucumber slices.

Nutritional Information (per serving)
Calories: 160
Fat total: 13.8g, saturated fat: 11.8g
Carbohydrates: 4.4g, dietary fiber: 1.1g
Sugars: 2.3g, protein: 6.2g

Popeye Breakfast Pie

Serves: 6
Prep Time: 20 minutes
Cooking Time: 35 minutes

Ingredients:
4 slices paleo-approved bacon, diced
45 ml (3 tablespoons) almond milk
6 eggs, whisked
1 red onion, chopped
1 cooked sweet potato, mashed
1 tomato, deseeded, chopped
15 ml (1 tablespoon) of jalapeños pepper, finely minced or 5 ml (1 teaspoon) of crushed dried chilies
1 bag of baby leaves spinach, grossly chopped
15 ml (1 tablespoon) flat leaf parsley (Italian parsley)
Sea salt and freshly ground pepper to taste

Directions:
1. Preheat oven to 180ºC/
2. 350°F. Lightly grease a baking pie dish with olive oil spray.
3. Combine well all ingredients in a mixing bowl. Season with salt and pepper.
4. Place batter into the pie dish.
5. Bake for 30 to 35 minutes or till golden browned.

Nutritional Information (per serving)
Calories: 330
Fat total: 24.3g, saturated fat: 15.2g
Carbohydrates: 15.9g, dietary fiber: 2.8g
Sugars: 6.0g, protein: 13.6g

You Could Eat Some All Day Pancakes

Serves: 4
Prep Time: 10 minutes
Cooking Time: 15 minutes

Ingredients:
6 eggs, lightly beaten
250 ml (1 cup) almond milk
250 ml (1 cup) almond flour
125 ml (½ cup) coconut flour
60 ml (¼ cup) grounded flaxseed
1 medium-sized, very ripe banana, mashed
30 ml (2 tablespoons) maple syrup
5 ml (1 teaspoon) vanilla
5 ml (1 teaspoon) apple cider vinegar
1 ml (¼ teaspoon) sea salt

30 ml (2 tablespoons) of coconut butter
Maple syrup, to drizzle or fresh fruits with raw honey

Directions:
1. Combine eggs, mashed banana, almond milk, maple syrup, vanilla, and vinegar in a large mixing bowl. Beat for 2-3 minutes until light and fluffy.
2. Mix all the dry ingredients in a bowl. Add gradually to the egg mixture and blend well, beating at low speed for 2-3 minutes. You can also use a food processor and blend all ingredients for 1-2 minutes on medium speed.
3. Heat a large non-stick frying pan, and melt the coconut butter. Spoon about 60 ml (1/4 cup) of this batter into the pan and cook for 2-3 minutes or until slightly golden. Flip and cook other side. Repeat until all batter is gone.
4. Sprinkle pancakes with maple syrup or fresh fruits with some raw honey.

Nutritional Information (per serving)
Calories: 311
Fat total: 24.6g, saturated fat: 8.5g
Carbohydrates: 14.2g, dietary fiber: 3.3g
Sugars: 7.2g, protein: 11.2g

Mammoth Breakfast Casserole

Serves: 4
Prep Time: 10 minutes
Cooking Time: 40 minutes

Ingredients:
6 strips paleo-approved bacon, diced

4 paleo approved pork breakfast sausages
6 eggs, whisked
1 Spanish onion, diced
1 red bell pepper, deseeded, diced
2 tomatoes, deseeded, diced
1 cup of asparagus, sliced
5 ml (1 teaspoon) of crushed hot chilies (or more if you like more hot)
5 ml (1 teaspoon) cumin
2.5 ml (½ teaspoon) dried oregano (or 1 tablespoon of fresh oregano, chopped)
2.5 ml (½ teaspoon) dried thyme (or 1 tablespoon of fresh thyme, chopped)
2.5 ml (½ teaspoon) dried basil (or 1 tablespoon of fresh basil)
125 ml (½ cup) coconut cream
Salt and freshly ground pepper to taste

Directions:
1. Preheat oven to 190ºC/375°F and lightly grease a square baking dish 8x8 with olive oil spray.
2. Heat a skillet on high. Cook the diced bacon for 5 minutes, stirring occasionally. Add onions and sauté for 1-2 minutes more until the onions are tender and fragrant. Remove from heat and let cool a few minutes.
3. In the meantime, in a large mixing bowl, combine all remaining ingredients, mix well. Add the bacon and onion. Season with salt and pepper to taste. Remove bacon and onion mixture into a bowl. Season with salt and pepper.
4. Pour the egg mixture in the baking dish.
5. Bake for 30 to 35 minutes or till golden browned and fluffy
6. Serve immediately with sliced tomatoes.

Nutritional Information (per serving)
Calories: 463
Fat total: 38.9g, Saturated fat: 22.9g
Carbohydrates: 8.4g, dietary fiber: 2.4g
Sugars: 4.8g, protein: 21.3g

Cocoa Almond Squares

Serves: 4
Prep Time: 5 minutes
Cooking Time: 18 minutes

Ingredients:
250 ml (2 cups) almond flour
30 ml (2 tablespoons) coconut flour
90 ml (6 tablespoons) cocoa powder
2.5 ml (½ teaspoon) sea salt
2 egg whites
60 ml (¼ cup) raw honey
15 ml (1 tablespoon) coconut oil

Directions
1. Preheat oven to 180°C/350°F.
2. In a medium bowl, add almond flour, coconut flour, cocoa powder, and salt. Mix well.
3. In another bowl, whisk egg whites until soft and foamy. Add honey and coconut oil, and combine well.
4. Mix the wet ingredients with the dry ingredients until a smooth dough is formed.
5. Roll out dough onto a piece of parchment paper. Sandwich it between two sheets and then using a sharp knife, slice into squares.

6. Bake for 15 to 18 minutes.
7. Serve with hot tea or coffee.

Nutritional Information (per serving)
Calories: 309
Fat total: 15.3g, saturated fat: 7.1g
Carbohydrates: 44.5g, dietary fiber: 5.2g
Sugars: 35.8g, protein: 6.9g

Glorious Morning Smoothie

Serves: 2
Prep Time: 10 minutes
Cooking Time: 0 minutes

Ingredients:
500 ml (2 cups) almond milk
1 orange, preferably without seed, peeled, and sectioned
1 grapefruit, medium size, peeled, and sectioned
375 ml (1½ cup) frozen mango pieces
1 tablespoon of raw honey (optional)

Instructions:
1. Place all the ingredients, except the ice, in a blender. Include the raw honey, if you like it sweeter. Blend until smooth. If it is too liquid, add ice cubes and pulse blend until desired consistency.

Nutritional Information (per serving)
Calories: 444
Fat total: 40.1g, saturated fat: 14.7g
Carbohydrates: 13.3g, dietary fiber: 5.6g
Sugars: 4.1g, protein: 14.2g

Caveman Breakfast Hash

Serves: 4
Prep Time: 15 minutes
Cooking Time: 25 minutes

Ingredients:
For the sausage patties
450 g (1 pound) of ground pork or veal
1-2 garlic cloves, minced
2.5 ml (½ teaspoon) jalapeños, minced or 1 ml (¼ teaspoon)
crushed hot chilies flakes
2.5 ml (½ teaspoon) dry thyme
2.5 ml (½ teaspoon) dry rosemary
1 ml (¼ teaspoon) fennel seeds
1 egg
Sea salt and freshly ground pepper to taste

For the hash (all ingredients to be chopped should be about the same size)
4 paleo-approved bacon strip, diced
4 breakfast sausages, homemade or paleo approved, diced
4 eggs
1 tablespoon olive oil (optional)
1 yellow onion, diced

1 green bell pepper, diced
1 red bell pepper, diced
2 celery stalks, diced
1 sweet potato, diced
1 zucchini, diced
2 garlic cloves, minced
1 tablespoon jalapeños pepper, minced
Sea salt and fresh ground pepper to taste

Directions
Pre-heat the oven at 200ºC/400 F.

For the sausage patties:

1. Place all the ingredients in a mixing bowl and combine well. Let rest and cover with a plastic wrap for at least 30 minutes. Form equal sized patties.
2. In a large frying pan, heat some olive oil on high heat. Fry the patties until well done, about 3-4 minutes on each side on medium-high heat. Do not press down too much on the patties while cooking or they will harden.

For the hash

1. In a large skillet, cook the bacon on high heat for 2-3 minutes until golden. Add onions and garlic, and continue cooking on medium heat for 2-3 minutes. Add sweet potatoes, cook for 5-6 minutes until the bacon is cooked. Add remaining ingredients. Cook for an additional 5-6 minutes or until all the vegetables are tender-crisp. Season with salt and pepper to taste. Remove the pan from heat and reserve.
2. In another frying pan, cook the eggs sunny side up until done. Season with salt and pepper to taste
3. Spoon ¼ of the hash on a plate, top with one sunny egg. Repeat for each serving.

Nutritional Information (per serving)

Calories: 444
Fat total: 40.1g, saturated fat: 14.7g
Carbohydrates: 13.3g, dietary fiber: 5.6g
Sugars: 4.1g, protein: 14.2g

Breakfast Paleo Waffles

Serves: 4 - Yields 4-5 waffles depending on waffle maker size
Prep Time: 15 minutes
Cooking Time: 15 minutes

Ingredients:
1 cup almond flour
30 ml (2 tablespoons) coconut flour
½ teaspoon baking soda
¼ teaspoon cinnamon
¼ teaspoon salt
4 eggs, separated
15 ml (1 tablespoon) olive oil
¼ cup coconut milk
¼ cup unsweetened organic applesauce or mashed ripe banana
(depends on your taste)
1 teaspoon vanilla
Fresh fruits for garnish or unsweetened organic applesauce or
maple syrup

Instructions:
1. Lightly grease the waffle maker with coconut butter and
   preheat.
2. In a bowl, beat egg whites on high speed for about 3
   minutes, until they form stiff peaks.

3. In a bowl, mix flour, baking soda, cinnamon, and salt. In another bowl, whisk egg yolks, milk, applesauce, or mashed banana, vanilla and oil.
4. Add flour mixture to the wet mixture and combine well. Fold in ¼ of the egg whites and mix well. Add another ¼ of egg whites, and gently fold it into the batter. Repeat twice. You should have a light and fluffy batter.
5. Place ⅓ cup to ½ cup of the batter in the greased waffle iron. Close gently and cook until golden browned.
6. Top with fresh fruits or unsweetened organic applesauce or a maple syrup drizzle

Nutritional Information (per serving)
Calories: 444
Fat total: 40.1g, saturated fat: 14.7g
Carbohydrates: 13.3g, dietary fiber: 5.6g
Sugars: 4.1g, protein: 14.2g

Hungry Man Steak and Bacon Hash

Serves: 4
Prep Time: 30 minutes
Cooking Time: 25 minutes

Ingredients:
4 paleo-approved bacon strips, chopped
½ pound of thinly sliced beef strips such as sirloin, chopped
4 eggs
1 tablespoon olive oil (optional)
½ cup chopped onions

½ cup green bell pepper chopped
½ cup red bell pepper, chopped
1 sweet potato, cubed
1 zucchini, cubed
2 garlic cloves, minced
1 tablespoon jalapeños pepper, minced
Sea salt & fresh ground pepper to taste

Instructions:

1. Pre-heat the oven at 200°C/400 F

2. In a large frying pan, cook the bacon for 2-3 minutes until golden on high heat. Add onions and garlic, and continue cooking on medium heat for 2-3 minutes. Add the beef and sweet potatoes, cook for 5-6 minutes until the meat is cooked. Add remaining ingredients and cook for an additional 10 minutes or until all the vegetables are tender. Season with salt and pepper to taste. Remove the pan from heat.
3. In another frying pan, cook the eggs sunny side up until done. Season with salt and pepper to taste
4. Spoon ¼ of the meat and vegetable mix on a plate, top with one sunny egg. Repeat for each serving.

Nutritional Information (per serving)

Calories: 444
Fat total: 40.1g, saturated fat: 14.7g,
Carbohydrates: 13.3g, dietary fiber: 5.6g
Sugars: 4.1g, protein: 14.2g

No-Crust Mini Bacon Quiches

Serves: 8
Prep Time: 15 minutes
Cooking Time: 25 minutes

Ingredients:
4 paleo-approved bacon strips, chopped
6 eggs
2 tablespoons olive oil (optional)
½ cup chopped onions
½ cup green bell pepper chopped
½ cup red bell pepper, chopped
Sea salt and fresh ground pepper to taste
Coconut butter or olive oil for greasing
Paprika to sprinkle

Instructions:
1. Pre-heat the oven at 190ºC/375 Fº.
2. In a large frying pan, cook the bacon for 5 minutes until golden brown on medium-high heat. Add onions, cooking on medium heat for 2 minutes. Add peppers, cook for 2 minutes, season with salt and pepper to taste. Remove the pan from heat and let cool a few minutes.
3. In the meantime, whisk the eggs vigorously for 2-3 minutes until very fluffy, then add the vegetables and bacon to the eggs and combine well. Season with salt and pepper to taste.
4. Grease generously a muffin pan with olive oil or coconut butter. Fill ¾ of each muffin hole with the egg mixture
5. Bake the egg muffins in the preheated oven for 10-12 minutes or until golden brown. Let cool for 5-10 minutes before unmolding, sprinkle with paprika. Serve hot with slices of tomatoes.

Nutritional Information (per serving)

Calories: 444
Fat total: 40.1g, saturated fat: 14.7g
Carbohydrates: 13.3g, dietary fiber: 5.6g
Sugars: 4.1g, protein: 14.2g

Pumpkin Breakfast Pancakes

Serves: 2
Prep Time: 5 minutes
Cooking Time: 10 minutes

Ingredients:
30 ml (2 teaspoons) coconut oil
250 ml (1 cup) pumpkin, pre-boiled and mashed
15 ml (1 tablespoon) almond butter
5 ml (1 teaspoon) pumpkin pie spice
5 ml (1 teaspoon) cinnamon
5 ml (1 teaspoon) vanilla extract
2 eggs, lightly beaten
15 ml (1 tablespoon) toasted almonds, chopped
15 ml (1 tablespoon) maple syrup

Directions:
1. Mash pumpkin in a bowl. Mix with almond butter.
2. Add in pumpkin pie spice, cinnamon, and vanilla extract and mix well.
3. Stir in eggs and whisk to combine well.
4. Heat oil in a nonstick skillet on medium heat.
5. Add 3 heaping tablespoons of batter into the pan and cook pancake for 2-3 minutes or until nicely golden. Flip and cook the other side and repeat until all batter is gone.

6. Serve on a plate, sprinkled with toasted nuts and drizzled with maple syrup.

Nutritional Information (per serving)
Calories: 258
Fat total: 16.1g, saturated fat: 6.2g
Carbohydrates: 21.2g, dietary fiber: 5.0g
Sugars: 10.9g, protein: 9.4g

Poblano Pepper Omelet

Serves: 2
Prep Time: 10 minutes
Cooking Time: 10 minutes

Ingredients:
30 ml (2 tablespoons) coconut oil
4 eggs
1 avocado, sliced
1 poblano pepper, sliced
1 onion, chopped
1 tomato, chopped
Salt and pepper to taste

Directions:
1. Crack eggs in a bowl, season with salt and pepper and whisk.
2. Heat oil in a frying pan.
3. Pour eggs in the pan. Tilt the pan to spread the eggs evenly. Top with avocado slices, poblano pepper, onion, and tomato.

4. Cook for 5 minutes or until set and slightly golden. Flip and cook the other side for 5 more minutes or until lightly golden. Fold into half and serve on a plate.

Nutritional Information (per serving)
Calories: 317
Fat total: 28.0g, saturated fat: 11.1g
Carbohydrates: 6.3g, dietary fiber: 5.7g
Sugars: 3.7g, protein: 9.5g

Jalapeño Scrambled Eggs with Cherry Tomatoes

Serves: 3
Prep Time: 5 minutes
Cooking Time: 15 minutes

Ingredients:
4 large eggs
2 egg whites
Salt and black pepper, to taste
5 ml (1 teaspoon) dried thyme
45 ml (3 tablespoons) almond butter
250 ml (1 cup) cherry tomatoes, halved
2 small jalapeños, seeded and chopped
4 scallions, chopped

Directions
1. In a bowl, add eggs, egg whites, salt, black pepper, and thyme and whisk well.
2. Melt butter in a frying pan over medium-high heat.
3. Add tomatoes and jalapeños, and cook for 2 to 3 minutes.

41

4. Add egg mixture and cook for 4 to 5 minutes until eggs are done completely, stirring occasionally.
5. Stir in scallions and cook for 1 to 2 minutes.

Nutritional Information (per serving)
Calories: 227
Fat total: 15.9g, saturated fat: 3.0g
Carbohydrates: 7.7g, dietary fiber: 2.1g
Sugars: 2.8g, protein: 15.2g

Peachy Pancakes

Serves: 2
Prep Time: 5 minutes
Cooking Time: 10 minutes

Ingredients:
250 ml (1 cup) peaches, chopped
2 eggs
60 ml (¼ cup) coconut milk
1 ml (¼ teaspoon) vanilla extract
15 ml (1 tablespoon) ground almond
30 ml (2 tablespoons) coconut flour
45 ml (3 tablespoons) ground flax seed
Pinch of cinnamon
Pinch of salt
30 ml (2 tablespoons) coconut oil

Directions
1. Lightly whisk eggs in a bowl, and add peaches.
2. Mix in coconut milk and vanilla extract and continue whisking.

3. In another bowl, mix together ground almond, coconut flour, flax seed, cinnamon, and salt.
4. Gradually add this mixture into eggs, and combine well using a fork.
5. Heat coconut oil in a nonstick frying pan. Spoon 30 ml (2 tablespoons) of this batter into the pan and flatten it using the backside of spoon.
6. Cook for 2-3 minutes or until slightly golden. Flip and cook other side, and repeat until all batter is gone. Serve in a plate topped with peach slices.

Nutritional Information (per serving)
Calories: 350
Fat total: 28.6g, saturated fat: 19.5g
Carbohydrates: 14.8g, dietary fiber: 8.9g
Sugars: 9.0g, protein: 8.9g

Mexican Scramble

Serves: 2
Prep Time: 10 minutes
Cooking Time: 15 minutes

Ingredients:
30 ml (2 tablespoons) coconut oil
1 medium onion, chopped
5 cloves garlic, minced
1 red bell pepper, deseeded, julienne
1 jalapeño pepper, deseeded, julienne
125 ml (½ cup) tomatoes, chopped
5 ml (1 teaspoon) cumin
2 large eggs

Seasons with salt and pepper
30 ml (2 tablespoons) parsley, chopped

Directions:
1. Heat oil in a large frying pan.
2. Stir in onion and garlic and cook for few minutes until little browned.
3. Add red bell pepper, jalapeño, and tomatoes and continue to cook until the vegetables are tender.
4. Sprinkle with cumin and salt.
5. Crack eggs in a bowl and season with salt and pepper.
6. Pour eggs in the frying pan.
7. Cook for 5 minutes or until slightly golden. Flip and cook other side until eggs are done.
8. Sprinkle with parsley and serve.

Nutritional Information (per serving)
Calories: 254
Fat total: 19.2g, saturated fat: 13.4g
Carbohydrates: 14.0g, dietary fiber: 3.4g
Sugars: 6.4g, protein: 8.6g

SNACK RECIPES
Healthy Granola Bars

Serves: 2
Prep Time: 5 minutes
Cooking Time: 15 minutes
Refrigerating time: 1 hour

Ingredients:
30 ml (2 tablespoons) pumpkin seeds
30 ml (2 tablespoons) poppy seeds
30 ml (2 tablespoons) sunflower seeds
30 ml (2 tablespoons) sesame seeds
30 ml (2 tablespoons) almonds, sliced
60 ml (4 tablespoons) freshly squeezed orange juice
15 ml (1 tablespoon) coconut oil
30 ml (2 tablespoons) raw honey

Directions:
1. Preheat oven to 180°C/350°F. Lightly grease a baking dish with olive oil.
2. Combine all ingredients in a bowl and seasons with salt and pepper.
3. Spread batter over a baking dish.
4. Bake for 10 to 15 minutes or until golden browned. Remove from oven and let it cool.
5. Cut into bars and refrigerate for at least 1 hour until set before serving.

Nutritional Information (per serving)
Calories: 333
Fat total: 23.6g, saturated fat: 8.1g,
Carbohydrates: 28.1g, dietary fiber: 3.4g
Sugars: 21.5g, protein: 7.4g

Paleo Beef Jerky

Serves: 2
Prep Time: 10 minutes
Marinating Time: 2 hours or overnight
Cooking Time: 4 hours

Ingredients:
225 g (½ pound) flank steak
30 ml (2 tablespoons) Coconut Amino
1 garlic clove, minced
2.5 ml (½ teaspoon) smoked paprika
2.5 ml (½ teaspoon) chipotle powder
2.5 ml (½ teaspoon) onion powder
2.5 ml (½ teaspoon) ginger powder
2.5 ml (½ teaspoon) salt
2.5 ml (½ teaspoon) black pepper

Directions:
1. Preheat the oven to 60°C/170°F. Lightly grease a baking dish.
2. Combine all ingredients in a bowl and mix together.
3. Leave marinated for at least 2 hours or overnight.
4. Put steak on the baking dish and bake for 3 to 4 hours.

Nutritional Information (per serving)
Calories: 234
Fat total: 9.6g, saturated fat: 3.9g
Carbohydrates: 3.1g, dietary fiber: 0.5g
Sugars: 0.0g, protein: 31.9g

Spicy Nuts

Serves: 2
Prep Time: 5 minutes
Cooking Time: 0 minutes

Ingredients:
5 ml (1 teaspoon) coconut oil
60 ml (¼ cup) pecans, toasted
60 ml (¼ cup) almonds, toasted
60 ml (¼ cup) walnuts, toasted
2.5 ml (½ teaspoon) chili powder
1 ml (¼ teaspoon) cumin
Pinch of salt and pepper

Directions:

1. Toss all ingredients in a mixing bowl and season with salt and pepper.

Nutritional Information (per serving)
Calories: 281
Fat total: 27.2g, saturated fat: 3.8g
Carbohydrates: 6.5g, dietary fiber: 4.1g
Sugars: 1.2g, protein: 7.7g

Watermelon & Kiwi with Fresh Herbs

Serves: 2
Prep Time: 10 minutes
Cooking Time: 0 minutes

Ingredients:
1000 ml (4 cups) watermelon
1 kiwi, chopped
2.5 ml (½ teaspoon) fresh oregano, chopped
2.5 ml (½ teaspoon) fresh cilantro, chopped
2.5 ml (½ teaspoon) fresh mint leaves
2.5 ml (½ teaspoon) fresh basil leaves, chopped
2.5 ml (½ teaspoon) fresh parsley, chopped
0.5 ml (⅛ teaspoon) salt
Pinch of ground black pepper

Directions:
1. Toss all ingredients in a mixing bowl and season with salt and pepper.

Nutritional Information (per serving)
Calories: 116
Fat total: 0.7g, saturated fat: 0.0g
Carbohydrates: 28.9g, dietary fiber: 2.6g
Sugars: 22.3g, protein: 2.4g

Ginger Green Smoothie

Serves: 1
Prep Time: 10 minutes
Cooking Time: 0 minutes

Ingredients:
1 cup of frozen mango pieces
1 apple, peeled, and core removed
¼ teaspoon, fresh ginger
30 ml (2 tablespoons) flax seeds
1 kale leave
60 ml (¼ cup) spinach
15 ml (1 tablespoon) lemon juice
250 ml (1 cup) water

Directions:
1. Place all the ingredients in blender or juicer and pulse until smooth.
2. Serve and enjoy!

Nutritional Information (per serving)
Calories: 163
Fat total: 2.4g, saturated fat: 0.0g
Carbohydrates: 31.6g, dietary fiber: 8.8g
Sugars: 17.3g, protein: 4.9g

Tropical Delight Fruit Bowl

Serves: 2
Prep Time: 10 minutes
Cooking Time: 0 minutes

Ingredients:
125 ml (½ cup) strawberries, chopped
1 yellow banana, peeled and sliced
125 ml (½ cup) mango chunks
1 kiwi, chopped

Directions:
1. Combine all the fruits in a bowl and serve.

Nutritional Information (per serving)
Calories: 121
Fat total: 0.5g, saturated fat: 0.0g
Carbohydrates: 29.8g, dietary fiber: 6.5g
Sugars: 19.4g, protein: 1.6g

Seasoned Seaweeds

Serves: 2
Prep Time: 5 minutes
Cooking Time: 5 minutes

Ingredients:
3 nori sheets, cut into small pieces
30 ml (2 tablespoons) coconut oil
15 ml (1 tablespoon) sesame oil
Pinch of salt

Directions:
1. Preheat oven to 180°C/350°F.
2. Toss nori sheets in a bowl with oils and sprinkle with salt.
3. Bake for 5 minutes.
4. Serve and enjoy.

Nutritional Information (per serving)
Calories: 192
Fat total: 20.4g, saturated fat: 12.7g
Carbohydrates: 1.5g, dietary fiber: 0.0g
Sugars: 0.0g, protein: 1.5g

S. & B. Smoothie

Serves: 2
Prep Time: 10 minutes
Cooking Time: 0 minutes

Ingredients:
250 ml (1 cup) watermelon, chunks
1 banana, sliced
250 ml (1 cup) strawberries
125 ml (½ cup) coconut milk

Directions:
1. Place all the ingredients in food processor, and blend until smooth and creamy. Serve and enjoy!

Nutritional Information (per serving)
Calories: 217
Fat total: 14.7g, saturated fat: 12.7g
Carbohydrates: 23.5g, dietary fiber: 4.1g
Sugars: 14.5g, protein: 2.6g

Apple Chips

Serves: 2
Prep Time: 5 minutes
Cooking Time: 30 minutes

Ingredients:
2 apples, thinly sliced crosswise
1 cinnamon stick
1000 ml (4 cups) fresh apple juice
Pinch of salt and pepper
Cinnamon to taste

Directions:
1. Preheat the oven to 180°C/350°F. Lightly grease a baking dish.
2. Combine all ingredients in a mixing bowl and season with salt and pepper. Sprinkle cinnamon to taste.
3. Cover and marinate overnight.
4. Spread apple on a baking dish.
5. Bake for 25 to 30 minutes or until browned.

Nutritional Information (per serving)
Calories: 214
Fat total: 0.3g, saturated fat: 0.0g
Carbohydrates: 54.9g, dietary fiber: 5.2g
Sugars: 46.0g, protein: 0.2g

Carrot Smoothie

Serves: 2
Prep Time: 10 minutes
Cooking Time: 0 minutes

Ingredients:
250 ml (1 cup) almond milk
250 ml (1 cup) carrots, chopped
1 banana, sliced
250 ml (1 cup) spinach
30 ml (2 tablespoons) cherries
15 ml (1 tablespoon) raw honey

Directions:
1. Place all the ingredients into a food processor and blend until smooth and creamy. Serve and enjoy!

Nutritional Information (per serving)
Calories: 392
Fat total: 29.0g, saturated fat: 25.5g
Carbohydrates: 36.0g, dietary fiber: 6.1g
Sugars: 22.5g, protein: 4.4g

Spicy Cauliflower

Serves: 2
Prep Time: 5 minutes
Cooking Time: 20 minutes

Ingredients:
1 head cauliflower, chopped
2.5 ml (½ teaspoon) cayenne pepper
½ tablespoon paprika
2.5 ml (½ teaspoon) red pepper flakes
2.5 ml (½ teaspoon) dried oregano
Pinch of salt and ground black pepper
60 ml (4 tablespoons) coconut oil

Directions:
1. Preheat the oven to 190°C/375°F.
2. Toss all ingredients in a mixing bowl. Season with salt and pepper.
3. Place on the baking dish in preheated oven.
4. Bake for 15 to 20 minutes until cauliflower is tender.

Nutritional Information (per serving)
Calories: 277
Fat total: 27.8g, saturated fat: 23.6g
Carbohydrates: 8.7g, dietary fiber: 4.4g
Sugars: 3.5g, protein: 3.0g

Spicy Fruit Salad

Serves: 2
Prep Time: 10 minutes
Cooking Time: 0 minutes

Ingredients:
1 apple, peeled and sliced
125 ml (½ cup) strawberries, chopped
125 ml (½ cup) orange, peeled and sliced
2.5ml (½ teaspoon) ground cinnamon
1 pinch cardamom

Directions:
1. Combine all the fruits in a bowl, sprinkle spices and serve.

Nutritional Information (per serving)
Calories: 83
Fat total: 0.2g, saturated fat: 0.0g
Carbohydrates: 21.1g, dietary fiber: 6.3g
Sugars: 15.4g, protein: 0.7g

Kale Chips

Serves: 2
Prep Time: 5 minutes
Cooking Time: 15 minutes

Ingredients:
1000 ml (4 cups) kale, remove stems and chop leaves
30 ml (2 tablespoons) coconut oil, melted
1ml (¼ teaspoon) salt
2.5ml (1/2 teaspoon) smoked paprika

Directions:
1. Preheat oven to 180°C/350°F.
2. Toss kale in a bowl with oil and sprinkle with salt.
3. Place kale leaves on a baking sheet, cover sheet with a parchment paper. Bake for 10 to 15 minutes or until kale is crispy.

Nutritional Information (per serving)
Calories: 36
Fat total: 2.5g, saturated fat: 2.0g
Carbohydrates: 3.4g, dietary fiber: 0.7g
Sugars: 0.0g, protein: 1.1g

Fresh Berry Cereal

Serves: 2
Prep Time: 5 minutes
Cooking Time: 0 minutes

Ingredients:
60 ml (¼ cup) strawberries
60 ml (¼ cup) blackberries
60 ml (¼ cup) blueberries
60 ml (¼ cup) raspberries
60 ml (¼ cup) unsweetened pomegranate seeds
60 ml (¼ cup) dried raisins, unsweetened
60 ml (¼ cup) almonds, chopped
125 ml (½ cup) almond milk

Directions:
1. Put all ingredients in a bowl and mix till well combined.
2. Serve and enjoy.

Nutritional Information (per serving)
Calories: 298
Fat total: 20.5g, saturated fat: 13.1g
Carbohydrates: 28.0g, dietary fiber: 7.2g
Sugars: 14.6g, protein: 5.2g

Banana Chips

Serves: 2
Prep Time: 5 minutes
Cooking Time: 30 minutes

Ingredients:
2 bananas cut into thin slices of about 2 mm (⅛ inch)
30 ml (2 tablespoons) lemon juice
30 ml (2 tablespoons) ground nutmeg

Directions
1. Preheat oven to 150°C/300° F. Line a baking sheet with parchment paper.
2. In a medium bowl, add all ingredients and mix well.
3. Spread banana slices evenly over the baking sheet in a single layer. Make sure banana slices are at least ½ inch apart.
4. Bake for 30 minutes or until banana slices are nicely golden in color.
5. Remove from oven, let cool a little and then serve.

Nutritional Information (per serving)
Calories: 145
Fat total: 3.1g, saturated fat: 2.0g
Carbohydrates: 30.8g, dietary fiber: 4.6g
Sugars: 16.7g, protein: 1.8g

Fruity Cinnamon Smoothie

Serves: 1
Prep Time: 5 minutes
Cooking Time: 0 minutes

Ingredients:
125 ml (½ cup) almond milk
60 ml (¼ cup) water
1 peach, pitted, peeled and sliced
1 banana, sliced
5 ml (1 teaspoon) raw honey
15 ml (1 tablespoon) cinnamon
4 ice cubes

Directions:
1. Place all the ingredients in a food processor and blend until smooth and creamy. Serve and enjoy!

Nutritional Information (per serving)
Calories: 457
Fat total: 29.3g, at saturated: 25.5g
Carbohydrates: 54.2g, dietary fiber: 4.9g
Sugars: 22.5g, protein: 2.6g

Primal Trail Mix

Serves: 2
Prep Time: 10 minutes
Cooking Time: 0 minutes

Ingredients:
60 ml (¼ cup) unsweetened dried apricots
60 ml (¼ cup) unsweetened dried banana, slices
60 ml (¼ cup) unsweetened raisins
125 ml (½ cup) dried unsweetened cranberries
125 ml (½ cup) raw sunflower seeds
60 ml (¼ cup) raw pumpkin seeds
60 ml (¼ cup) raw almonds, chopped

Directions:
1. Place all the ingredients in a bowl and mix together.
2. Serve and enjoy!

Nutritional Information (per serving)
Calories: 392
Fat total: 22.8g, saturated fat: 5.0g
Carbohydrates: 42.7g, dietary fiber: 6.2g
Sugars: 21.2g, protein: 11.4g

St. Patrick Day Smoothie

Serves: 1
Prep Time: 5 minutes
Cooking Time: 0 minutes

Ingredients:
125 ml (½ cup) mango pieces (fresh or frozen)
250 ml (1 cup) baby spinach leaves
125 ml (½ cup) unsweetened almond milk
15 ml (1 tablespoon) grounded flaxseeds
60 ml (¼ cup) water
15 ml (1 tablespoon) raw honey
125 ml (½ cup) ice cubes (optional)

Directions:
1. Place all the ingredients in a food processor and blend until smooth and creamy.
2. Serve and enjoy!

Nutritional Information (per serving)
Calories: 144
Fat total: 4.1, saturated fat: 0
Carbohydrates: 21.1g, dietary fiber: 3.2g
Sugars: 0.1g, protein: 2.9

Minty Fruits Salad

Serves: 2
Prep Time: 5minutes
Cooking Time: 0 minutes

Ingredients:
125 ml (½ cup) lime juice
60 ml (4 tablespoons) mint leaves, chopped
1 banana, sliced
½ apple, sliced
30 ml (2 tablespoons) grapes
125 ml (½ cup) mango chunks
30 ml (2 tablespoons) strawberries, chopped
1 kiwi, peeled and cut into 1 inches chunks
Pinch of salt

Directions:
1. In a food processor, add lime juice and mint, and pulse until smooth.
2. Combine all the fruits in a bowl, sprinkle with a pinch of salt, and serve drizzled with lime juice mixture.

Nutritional Information (per serving)
Calories: 163
Fat total: 0.6g, saturated fat: 0.0g
Carbohydrates: 42.3g, dietary fiber: 6.6g
Sugars: 25.0g, protein: 2.2g

Blueberry & Spinach Smoothie

Serves: 2
Prep Time: 5 minutes
Cooking Time: 0 minutes

Ingredients:
250 ml (1 cup) blueberries
1 banana, sliced
250 ml (1 cup) spinach leaves
125 ml (½ cup) coconut milk
15 ml (1 tablespoon) raw honey

Directions:
1. Place all the ingredients into a food processor, and blend until smooth and creamy. Serve and enjoy!

Nutritional Information (per serving)
Calories: 267
Fat total: 14.8g, saturated fat: 12.8g
Carbohydrates: 36.5g, dietary fiber: 5.0g
Sugars: 25.1g, protein: 3.0g

Pumpkin Pie Spice with Sweet Potato

Serves: 2
Prep Time: 5 minutes
Cooking Time: 15 minutes

Ingredients:
2 sweet potatoes, pre-cooked and peeled
125 ml (½ cup) coconut milk
5 ml (1 teaspoon) pumpkin pie spice
5 ml (1 teaspoon) cinnamon
15 ml (1 tablespoon) raw honey
15 ml (1 tablespoon) butter
Pinch of salt and pepper

Directions:
1. Preheat the oven to 180°C/350°F. Lightly grease a pie dish.
2. Combine all ingredients in a mixing bowl, and season with salt and pepper.
3. Pour batter in pie dish.
4. Bake for 15 minutes or until browned.

Nutritional Information (per serving)
Calories: 404
Fat total: 20.4g, saturated fat: 16.4g
Carbohydrates: 55.3g, dietary fiber: 8.2g
Sugars: 11.5g, protein: 3.9g

LUNCH RECIPES
Salmon, Spinach & Apple Salad

Serves: 2
Prep Time: 15 minutes
Cooking Time: 30 minutes

Ingredients:
225 g (½ pound) salmon fillets

For salad
250 ml (1 cup) baby spinach
125 ml (½ cup) lettuce
125 ml (½ cup) cabbage, shredded
1 tart apple such as Granny Smith, sliced

For dressing
30 ml (2 tablespoons) olive oil
30 ml (2 tablespoons) apple cider vinegar
1 large shallot, minced
Salt and black pepper, to taste

Directions:
1. Preheat the oven to 180ºC/350° F.
2. Place salmon fillet on a baking dish. Season with salt and pepper.
3. Add some water to cover the fish. Cover with foil.
4. Bake for 10 minutes. Remove from oven and set aside.
5. In a large bowl, add salad ingredients and mix.
6. In another bowl, add all dressing ingredients and whisk till well combined.
7. Pour dressing over salad and toss to coat.
8. Serve salad with baked fish fillets.

Nutritional Information (per serving)
Calories: 334
Fat total: 21.1g, saturated fat: 3.0g
Carbohydrates: 15.6g, dietary fiber: 3.1g
Sugars: 10.4g, protein: 22.9g

Sautéed Coconut Chicken

Serves: 3-4
Prep Time: 10 minutes
Cooking Time: 20 minutes

Ingredients:
450 g (1 pound) boneless and skinless chicken breasts cut in strips
60 ml (¼ cup) coconut flour
60 ml (¼ cup) shredded coconut, organic, unsweetened
0.5 ml (⅛ teaspoon) sea salt
1 egg
30 ml (2 tablespoons) coconut oil

Directions:
1. Whisk together coconut flour, shredded coconut, and salt in a medium bowl.
2. In another bowl, beat egg.
3. Dip chicken breast strips in the egg and then into the flour mixture.
4. Heat oil in a frying pan over medium-high heat.
5. Place chicken in the pan and cook until golden brown from both sides.
6. Remove from the pan and serve in a plate.

Nutritional Information (per serving)
Calories: 298
Fat total: 15.1g, saturated fat: 10.6g
Carbohydrates: 6.5g, dietary fiber: 3.9g
Sugars: 1.2g, protein: 34.3g

The Big Salad

Serves: 4
Prep Time: 20 minutes
Cooking Time: 0 minute

Ingredients
For Salad
300 grams (2 cups) cooked chicken breast, chopped
2 liters (8 cups) spring mix lettuce
1 English cucumber, diced
12 cherry tomatoes
1 avocado, diced
60 ml (¼ cup) dry unsweetened cranberries
60 ml (¼ cup) chopped raw pecans or any favorite nuts
Sea salt and freshly ground pepper to taste

For Dressing – yield approximately 425 ml (1⅔cup)
1 cup extra virgin, cold press olive oil
60 ml (¼ cup) red wine vinegar
15 ml (1 tablespoon) Dijon mustard
30 ml (2 tablespoons) raw honey
60 ml (¼ cup) fresh basil leaves

Directions:
1. Blend together until smooth all the ingredient of the dressing
2. In a large salad bowl, place all the salad ingredients, season with salt and pepper to taste, add some dressing to taste and mix well.

Nutritional Information (per serving)
Calories: 398
Fat total: 15.1g, saturated fat: 10.6g
Carbohydrates: 6.5g, dietary fiber: 3.9g
Sugars: 1.2g, protein: 34.3g

Paleo Pizza

Serves: 8
Prep Time: 10 minutes
Cooking Time: 55 minutes

Ingredients
For crust:
1000 ml (4 cups) almond flour
2 eggs
45 ml (3 tablespoons) olive oil
5 ml (1 teaspoon) garlic powder
1 ml (¼ teaspoon) baking soda
2.5 ml (1½ tablespoon) fresh rosemary, chopped

For toppings:
250 ml (1 cup) organic marinara sauce
485 g (1 pound) Italian paleo pork sausage, sliced
250 ml (1 cup) yellow summer squash, diced

3 scallions, chopped
15 ml (1 tablespoon) basil leaves
2 small tomatoes, diced
125 ml (½ cup) roasted red peppers, diced
15 ml (1 tablespoon) black olives, sliced
Salt to taste

Directions:
1. Preheat the oven to 180°C/350° F. Lightly grease a pizza pan.
2. Place all the crust ingredients in a food processor and pulse until a dough forms.
3. Form a ball with the dough using your hands. Place the ball in the center of greased pizza pan. Then press the dough using your hands, patting and shaping it into a circle. Bake for 20 minutes or until cooked. Remove from oven. Let it cool.
4. In a bowl, add sausages, squash, scallions, basil, tomatoes, red pepper, olives, and salt and mix till well combined.
5. Spread pizza base with marinara sauce. Top with sausage mixture.
6. Return to oven and bake again for 25 to 35 minutes or until top is lightly golden.

Nutritional Information (per serving)
Calories: 433
Fat total: 35.3g, saturated fat: 7.5g
Carbohydrates: 12.9g, dietary fiber: 4.9g
Sugars: 5.1g, protein: 18.7g

Macadamia Hummus with Vegetables

Serves: 4
Prep Time: 20 minutes
Refrigerating Time: 30-45 minutes

Ingredients:
750 ml (3 cups) macadamia nuts
60 ml (¼ cup) freshly squeezed lemon juice
60 ml (¼ cup) olive oil
2 garlic cloves, minced
2.5 ml (½ teaspoon) salt
125 ml (½ cup) water
500 ml (2 cups) of baby carrots
1 English cucumber, chopped into sticks
1 Sweet pepper, deseeded and sliced

Directions:
1. Place all the ingredients in food processor except carrots and cucumbers and blend until smooth and thick.
2. Place hummus in a bowl and refrigerate to chill for 30 to 45 minutes before serving. Will keep for up to a week in the refrigerator.
3. Serve with the cut vegetables.

Nutritional Information (per serving)
Calories: 419
Fat total: 40.7g, saturated fat: 6.5g
Carbohydrates: 15.7g, dietary fiber: 6.0g
Sugars: 3.9g, protein: 5.3g

Carrot Soup

Serves: 2
Prep Time: 15 minutes
Cooking Time: 30 minutes

Ingredients:
30 ml (2 tablespoons) coconut oil
2 bay leaves
1 onion, sliced
4 garlic cloves, minced
250 ml (1 cup) carrots, chopped
2 turnips, chopped
2 sweet potatoes, cubed
1 ml (¼ teaspoon) dried thyme
1000 ml (4 cups) chicken broth
30 ml (2 tablespoons) fresh chives, chopped
Sea salt and freshly ground pepper to taste

Directions:
1. Heat oil in a large soup pan.
2. Stir in bay leaves, onion, and garlic, and sauté for few minutes until fragrant and tender.
3. Add carrots, turnips, sweet potatoes, and dried thyme, and continue to cook until the vegetables are tender.
4. Add broth and bring to boil. Cover and cook for 15 to 20 minutes.
5. Discard bay leaves. Pour soup in a food processor and pulse until smooth.
6. Season with salt and pepper.
7. Return to soup pan and let it simmer for 5 minutes.
8. Put soup in a bowl, sprinkle with chives, and serve hot.

Nutritional Information (per serving)
Calories: 340
Fat total: 15.5g, saturated fat: 12.2g
Carbohydrates: 43.7g, dietary fiber: 8.5g
Sugars: 11.0g, protein: 8.7g

Grilled Chicken with Olive and Tomato Topping

Serves: 2
Prep Time: 5 minutes
Cooking Time: 10 minutes

Ingredients:

For topping:
30 ml (2 tablespoons) parsley, chopped
30 ml (2 tablespoons) basil sprigs
1 garlic clove
2 sundried tomatoes
30 ml (2 tablespoons) olives, pitted
60 ml (¼ cup) lemon juice

For Chicken
2 skinless and boneless chicken breasts
30 ml (2 tablespoons) coconut oil
1 ml (¼ teaspoon) salt

Directions:
1. Place all the topping ingredients in a food processor and blend until smooth. Set aside.
2. Preheat a grill pan to high.

3. Toss chicken in a bowl with oil and sprinkle with salt.
4. Place chicken on a grill pan over medium.
5. Grill for 5 minutes on each side, or until well cooked (to your desired doneness). Serve on a platter drizzled with topping.

Nutritional Information (per serving)
Calories: 338
Fat total: 17.9g, saturated fat: 12.6g
Carbohydrates: 32.1g, dietary fiber: 7.2g
Sugars: 21.0g, protein: 20.2g

Grilled Shrimps Salad

Serves: 2
Prep Time: 5 minutes
Cooking Time: 10 minutes

Ingredients:
225 g (½ pound) medium shrimp
30 ml (2 tablespoons) olive oil
15 ml (1 tablespoon) garlic, minced
Salt to taste
5 ml (1 teaspoon) red pepper flakes, crushed
30 ml (2 tablespoons) lemon juice
45 ml (3 tablespoons) fresh parsley, chopped
500ml (2 cups) mixed greens salad
2.5 ml (1 tablespoon) apple cider vinegar
7.5 ml (3 tablespoons) grapeseed oil

Directions:
1. Preheat a grill pan to high.
2. Toss shrimps in a bowl with oil and garlic and sprinkle with salt and red pepper flakes.
3. Place shrimps on a grill pan over medium.
4. Grill for 5 minutes on each side or until tender.
5. To prepare the dressing, mix vigorously grapeseed oil and vinegar in a salad bowl with a whisk. Season with salt and freshly ground pepper to taste and add the mixed greens. Combine well. Top with the shrimps.
6. Drizzled the lemon juice over the shrimps and sprinkled with parsley.

Nutritional Information (per serving)
Calories: 243
Fat total: 15.7g, saturated fat: 2.2g
Carbohydrates: 2.6g, dietary fiber: 0.6g
Sugars: 0.5g, protein: 25.0g

Broccoli & Pine Nuts Soup

Serves: 2
Prep Time: 5 minutes
Cooking Time: 30 minutes

Ingredients:
30 ml (2 tablespoons) coconut oil
1 onion, diced
1000 ml (4 cups) broccoli
750 ml (3 cups) vegetable broth
60 ml (¼ cup) pine-nuts

Directions:
1. Heat oil in a large pan.
2. Stir in onion and broccoli, cook for few minutes until broccoli is little tender.
3. Add broth and pine nuts and bring to a boil. Cover and cook medium low for 10 to 15 minutes.
4. Place soup in a food processor and pulse until smooth and thick.
5. Return to soup pan and let it simmer for 5 minutes.
6. Ladle soup in a serving bowl and serve hot.

Nutritional Information (per serving)
Calories: 312
Fat total: 22.4g, saturated fat: 12.8g
Carbohydrates: 14.1g, dietary fiber: 3.9g
Sugars: 5.2g, protein: 13.8g

Brussels Sprouts & Bacon with Tandoori Drumsticks

Serves: 4
Prep Time: 15 minutes
Cooking Time: 25 minutes

Ingredients:
15 ml (1 tablespoon) olive oil
2 slices paleo-approved bacon, diced
500 ml (2 cups) Brussels sprouts, trimmed and halved
1 onion, sliced
10 ml (2 teaspoons) freshly squeezed lemon juice
Salt and freshly ground pepper to taste

Directions:
1. Heat oil in a pan over medium heat.
2. Stir in bacon and cook for 4-5 minutes until bacon is a little browned, add onions and sauté for 2-3 minutes.
3. Add Brussels sprouts continue to cook for 15 more minutes, stirring occasionally, until sprouts are tender.
4. Drizzle lemon juice, season with salt and pepper.
5. Serve with left-over tandoori chicken drumsticks.

Nutritional Information (per serving – Brussels sprouts only)
Calories: 224
Fat total: 15.1g, saturated fat: 3.7g
Carbohydrates: 9.3g, dietary fiber: 2.8g
Sugars: 3.2g, protein: 9.1g

Delightful Vegetable Medley Soup

Serves: 2
Prep Time: 15 minutes
Cooking Time: 35 minutes

Ingredients:
30 ml (2 tablespoons) coconut oil
1 onion, diced
2 garlic cloves, chopped
5 ml (1 teaspoon) ginger, chopped
125 ml (½ cup) cauliflower, chopped
125 ml (½ cup) yellow squash, cubed
30 ml (2 tablespoons) celery, chopped
750 ml (3 cups) vegetable broth
Salt and pepper, to taste
15 ml (1 tablespoon) lemon juice

Directions:
1. Heat oil in a large pan over medium heat.
2. Sauté onion, garlic, and ginger for a few minutes or until tender and fragrant.
3. Add cauliflower, yellow squash, and celery, and cook for 5 minutes, stirring occasionally.
4. Add broth and bring to a boil on high heat. Bring heat down to medium, cover and cook for 15 to 20 minutes or until vegetables are tender. Remove from heat and cool a little.
5. Place soup in a food processor, and pulse until smooth and thick.
6. Return to soup pan, season, and let the soup simmer for 5 minutes until reheated.
7. Ladle soup into a soup bowl, drizzle with lemon juice and serve.

Nutritional Information (per serving)
Calories: 223
Fat total: 15.9g, saturated fat: 12.4g
Carbohydrates: 11.7g, dietary fiber: 2.6g
Sugars: 4.6g, protein: 0.4g

Paleo Prawns with Tomato Sauce

Serves: 2
Prep Time: 5 minutes
Cooking Time: 10 minutes

Ingredients:
30 ml (2 tablespoons) olive oil
1 red onion, chopped

1 cloves garlic, minced
225 g (½ pound) prawns
2 medium tomatoes, chopped
2.5 ml (½ teaspoon) cayenne pepper
5 ml (1 teaspoon) oregano
30 ml (2 tablespoons) celery, chopped
30 ml (2 tablespoons) capers
2.5 ml (½ teaspoon) sea salt
2.5 ml (½ teaspoon) black pepper

Directions:
1. Heat oil in a large frying pan.
2. Stir in onion and garlic, and cook for few minutes until fragrant and tender.
3. Add prawns and tomatoes, and cook for 6-7 minutes until prawns are tender.
4. Sprinkle with cayenne pepper, oregano, celery, and capers. Season with salt and pepper and serve.

Nutritional Information (per serving)
Calories: 309
Fat: 16.4g, Saturated fat: 2.7g
Carbohydrates: 13.7g, dietary fiber: 3.6g
Sugars: 5.7g, protein: 28.0g

Salmon & Asparagus Salad

Serves: 2
Prep Time: 10 minutes
Cooking Time: 5 minutes

Ingredients:
250 ml (1 cup) salmon, boiled and shredded
125 ml (½ cup) onion, chopped
125 ml (½ cup) celery, chopped
125 ml (½ cup) asparagus
125 ml (½ cup) cherry tomatoes, halved
30 ml (2 tablespoons) olive oil
Spring mix salad
Salt and pepper to taste

Directions:
1. Steam asparagus in boiling water for 5-6 minutes. Drain asparagus and immediately add to a bowl filled with cold water, to stop the cooking process.
2. Toss all ingredients in a mixing bowl, and season with salt and pepper.
3. Serve on a bed of spring mix salad.

Nutritional Information (per serving)
Calories: 267
Fat total: 19.6g, saturated fat: 2.8g
Carbohydrates: 6.3g, dietary fiber: 2.2g
Sugars: 3.3g, protein: 18.8g

Cucumber & Watermelon Salad

Serves: 2
Prep Time: 5minutes
Cooking Time: 0 minutes

Ingredients:
1 cucumber, diced
1000 ml (4 cups) watermelon, seeded and diced
15 ml (1 tablespoon) red onion, sliced thinly
60 ml (4 tablespoons) fresh mint leaves, minced
30 ml (2 tablespoons) balsamic vinegar
45 ml (3 tablespoons) coconut oil
Salt and freshly ground black pepper, to taste
30 ml (2 tablespoons) walnuts, chopped

Directions:
1. Toss all ingredients in a mixing bowl, and season with salt and pepper.
2. Sprinkle with walnuts and serve.

Nutritional Information (per serving)
Calories: 302
Fat total: 25.5g, saturated fat: 17.9g
Carbohydrates: 19.3g, dietary fiber: 2.8g
Sugars: 9.8g, protein: 4.2g

Mushroom Cream Soup

Serves: 3
Prep Time: 10 minutes
Cooking Time: 20 minutes

Ingredients:
30 ml (2 tablespoons) coconut oil
1 onion, chopped
1 garlic clove, minced
2 avocados, sliced
250 ml (1 cup) mushrooms, sliced
1 red sweet pepper, chopped
2 tomatoes, sliced
4 sprigs basil leaves
750 ml (3 cups) chicken stock
250 ml (1 cup) coconut cream
Salt and freshly ground black pepper to taste

Directions:
1. Heat oil in a pan.
2. Add onion and garlic, and cook for 3 to 4 minutes until tender.
3. Add avocado, mushrooms, red sweet pepper, tomatoes, and basil leaves, and continue to cook until the vegetables are tender.
4. Add water and bring to a boil. Cover and cook for 15 minutes.
5. Sprinkle with salt and pepper.
6. When cooked, cool a little, place the soup into a food processor, and blend until smooth and creamy.
7. Reheat, ladle in a soup bowl and serve.

Nutritional Information (per serving)
Calories: 389
Fat total: 35.6g, saturated fat: 10.7g
Carbohydrates: 20.8g, dietary fiber: 11.9g
Sugars: 15.6g, protein: 14.1g

Paleo Tuna Salad

Serves: 2
Prep Time: 5 minutes
Cooking Time: 0 minutes

Ingredients:
1 avocado, mashed
Juice of 1 lemon
1 can tuna, drained
15 ml (1 tablespoon) onion, chopped
15 ml (1 tablespoon) celery, chopped
15 ml (1 tablespoon) carrot, shredded
Salt and pepper to taste
1000 ml (4 cups) organic mix greens

Directions:
1. In a bowl, combine mashed avocados with lemon juice.
2. Add the rest of the ingredients (except the organic mix greens) and combine gently.
3. Season with salt and pepper.
4. Place mix greens onto a large plate, spoon tuna mixture on top, and serve.

Nutritional Information (per serving)
Calories: 380
Fat total: 27.0g, saturated fat: 3.7g
Carbohydrates: 3.3g, dietary fiber: 7.9g
Sugars: 2.1g, protein: 26.5g

Chicken, Tomato, Mint & Basil salad

Serves: 2
Prep Time: 10 minutes
Cooking Time: 0 minutes

Ingredients:
1 skinless and boneless precooked chicken breast
1 green bell pepper, deseeded, julienne
2 tomatoes, deseeded, sliced
30 ml (2 tablespoons) fresh basil, chopped
30 ml (2 tablespoons) fresh mint, chopped
10 ml (2 teaspoons) vinegar
10 ml (2 teaspoons) avocado oil
Salt and freshly ground black pepper

Directions:
1. Toss all ingredients in a mixing bowl and season with salt and pepper.

Nutritional Information (per serving)
Calories: 173
Fat total: 6.1g, saturated fat: 1.5g
Carbohydrates: 6.6g, dietary fiber: 2.6g
Sugars: 4.2g, protein: 21.7g

Quick and Easy Egg Salad Wrap

Serves: 2
Prep Time: 10 minutes
Cooking Time: 0

Ingredients:
4 hard-boiled eggs
60 ml (¼ cup) red onion, finely chopped
2.5 ml (½ teaspoon) of cayenne pepper
60 ml (¼ cup) celery, chopped
10 black or green olives, chopped
60 ml (¼ cup) seedless cucumber, chopped
30 ml (2 tablespoons) of Paleo mayonnaise (see recipe below or store bought paleo mayonnaise)
4 large lettuce leaves such as Boston bib or romaine for the wrap
Salt and pepper for seasoning

Directions:
1. Mix all the ingredients.
2. Spoon the egg mixture generously into the lettuce leaves
3. Serve with fresh cut vegetables such as tomatoes and bell pepper

Nutritional Information (per serving)
Calories: 310
Fat total: 15.3g, saturated fat: 8.2g
Carbohydrates: 8.3g, dietary fiber: 0.0g
Sugars: 6.3g, protein: 33.5g

Paleo Mayonnaise Recipe

Yield approx. 285 ml – 1⅛ cup

Ingredients

250ml (1 cup) olive oil (use regular olive oil or you can substitute for avocado or macadamia oil)
1 large egg yolk
15 ml (1 tablespoon) fresh lemon juice
5 ml (1 teaspoon) dry mustard
1 ml (1/4 teaspoon) sea salt
Fresh ground pepper to taste

Directions:
1. Mix together the yolk, lemon, and mustard in a blender.
2. Slowly start dripping all the olive oil in the blender on low speed. The mayonnaise will start to thicken. Blend until firm, and mayonnaise texture is obtained.
3. Add salt and fresh ground pepper to taste.
4. Refrigerate in an air-tight container. It can last for up to 2-3 weeks

Sautéed Leeks with Salmon

Serves: 2
Prep Time: 10 minutes
Cooking Time: 30 minutes

Ingredients:
30 ml (2 tablespoons) almond butter, separated
125 ml (½ cup) chopped leeks
30 ml (2 tablespoons) chopped celery
2 carrots, sliced
2 salmon fillets, cut into strips
30 ml (2 tablespoons) lemon juice
Salt and pepper to taste

Directions:
1. Melt half of the almond butter in a sauté pan over medium.
2. Stir in carrots, and cook for 5 minutes, stirring often. Add leeks and celery, and continue cooking for 5 minutes more or until carrots are crisply tender. Remove vegetables onto a plate, and set aside.
3. Heat remaining butter in the same pan, and add salmon. Let simmer, stirring occasionally, for 15 minutes until fish is cooked through. Add in sautéed vegetables, and stir for 2 minutes until vegetables are heated through.
4. Drizzle lemon juice, season with salt and pepper and serve.

Nutritional Information (per serving)
Calories: 380
Fat total: 20.4g, saturated fat: 2.6g
Carbohydrates: 12.3g, dietary fiber: 2.9g
Sugars: 4.2g, protein: 39.0g

Chicken & Spinach

Serves: 2
Prep Time: 10 minutes
Cooking Time: 15 minutes

Ingredients:
45 ml (3 tablespoons) coconut oil
1 skinless and boneless chicken breast, cut into strips
1 garlic clove, minced
1 onion, chopped
250 ml (1 cup) spinach, washed and chopped
Salt and freshly ground black pepper to taste
125 ml (½ cup) organic, unsweetened, shredded coconut

Directions:
1. Heat oil in a large frying pan.
2. Stir in chicken and garlic, and cook for 8 to 10 minutes until little browned.
3. Add onion and spinach, and continue to cook for 5 minutes until the vegetables are tender.
4. Season with salt and pepper. Sprinkle with coconut and serve.

Nutritional Information (per serving)
Calories: 334
Fat total: 28.6g, saturated fat: 23.8g
Carbohydrates: 9.0g, dietary fiber: 3.3g
Sugars: 3.5g, protein: 13.8g

Salmon Salad

Serves: 2
Prep Time: 15 minutes
Cooking Time: 0 minute

Ingredients:
250 ml (1 cup) salmon, steamed until done, shredded
2 cucumbers, peeled and chopped
1 onion, chopped
1 large diced tomato
1 avocado, chopped
30 ml (2 tablespoons) olive oil
30 ml (2 tablespoons) lemon juice
30 ml (2 tablespoons) fresh dill
125 ml (½ cup) Lettuce leaves, shredded
Pinch of salt and freshly ground black pepper

Directions:
1. Toss and combine well all ingredients in a salad bowl.
   Season with salt and pepper.
2. Serve and enjoy.

Nutritional Information (per serving)
Calories: 300
Fat total: 24.1g, saturated fat: 3.0g
Carbohydrates: 14.9g, dietary fiber: 7.4g
Sugars: 3.9g, Protein: 7.7g

Lemon Grilled Chicken

Serves: 2
Prep Time: 5 minutes
Cooking Time: 25 minutes

Ingredients:
2 chicken thighs
30 ml (2 tablespoons) coconut oil
Pinch of salt and freshly ground black pepper
30 ml (2 teaspoons) lemon juice
½ tablespoon lemon zest

Directions:
1. Preheat a grill pan to high.
2. Toss chicken in a bowl with oil, and sprinkle with salt and pepper.
3. Place chicken on a grill pan over medium.
4. Grill thighs for 10 minutes on each side, turning occasionally (every 2-3 minutes), until thighs are cooked through. Then bring heat to high, and grill for 4 minutes on both sides to obtain visible grill marks.
5. Serve on a platter drizzled with lemon juice and sprinkled with lemon zest.

Nutritional Information (per serving)
Calories: 385
Fat total: 24.0g, saturated fat: 14.6g
Carbohydrates: 0.7g, dietary fiber: 0.0g
Sugars: 0.0g, protein: 40.6g

DINNER RECIPES
Piri Piri Chicken

Serves: 8
Prep Time: 30 minutes
Cooking Time: 65 minutes
Marinade time: 4h00 up to 12h00

Ingredients:
2 whole organic chickens
2 tablespoons of Piri Piri spice mix
4 garlic cloves, minced
1 onion, diced
60 ml (¼ cup) freshly squeezed lemon juice
60 ml (¼cup) organic maple syrup
5 ml (1 teaspoon) sea salt
85 ml (⅓ cup) olive oil
30 ml (2 tablespoons) apple cider vinegar
Sea salt and fresh ground pepper to taste

Instructions:
1. Mix all the ingredients except the chickens in a food processor. Blend until you obtain a smooth marinade.
2. Place the chicken on a working surface, breast side down. With a large and sharp knife, cut open the back of the chicken so that it will flatten and open up. Turn the chicken over, and press firmly to flatten. Repeat for the second chicken.
3. In a large zip lock bag, place one chicken in with half of the marinade. Repeat with the second chicken. Refrigerate for a minimum of 4 hours and up to 12 hours.
4. Remove both chickens from the marinade, and place in a roasting oven pan. Place the chickens, breast side facing

up. Season with salt and pepper to taste. Reserve the marinade.

5. Place the excess marinade in a small saucepan, and cook on low heat for 20 minutes
6. Place the chickens on the middle rack, in pre-heated 400°F oven, and cook for 30 minutes.
7. After 30 minutes, take out the chicken, smear with some of the marinade on both sides, and cook for another 30 minutes.
8. Brush the breast side with the rest of the marinade, and broil for 5 minutes.
9. Cut the chicken in pieces, and serve with steamed vegetables of your choice.

Nutritional Information (per serving)
Calories: 444
Fat total: 40.1g, saturated fat: 14.7g
Carbohydrates: 13.3g, dietary fiber: 5.6g
Sugars: 4.1g, protein: 14.2g

Nutty Tilapia Fillets

Serves: 4
Prep Time: 15 minutes
Cooking Time: 10 minutes

Ingredients:
4 large Tilapia fillets
15 ml (1 tablespoon) black peppercorn
8 ml (½ tablespoon) fennel seeds
8 ml (½ tablespoon) smoked paprika
45 ml (3 tablespoons) coconut butter or grass-fed butter

125 ml (½ cup) of pecan
15 ml (1 tablespoon) fresh chopped flat leave parsley
Sea salt & fresh ground pepper to taste
1 lemon, sliced

Instructions:
1. Using a pestle and a mortar, crush and grind together peppercorn, fennel seeds, and paprika
2. Season both sides of the tilapia with the spices.
3. Using a frying pan, melt 2 tablespoons of the butter on medium heat. Add the fillets, and cook for 4 minutes, turn the tilapia over and cook for an additional 3 to 4 minutes until the fish is done.
4. Place your cooked fillets on a warm serving plate, and reserve.
5. In the same hot frying pan, add the rest of the butter and the pecans. Cook for about 1 minute. Add some lemon juice to taste, and mix well.
6. Place the lemony nuts on the fillets, sprinkle with the parsley, and serve with your favorite side vegetables and lemon slices.

Nutritional Information (per serving)
Calories: 444
Fat total: 40.1g, saturated fat: 14.7g
Carbohydrates: 13.3g, dietary fiber: 5.6g
Sugars: 4.1g, protein: 14.2g

Tandoori Chicken Drumsticks & Mango Chutney

Serves: 8
Prep Time: 45 minutes
Cooking Time: 30 minutes
Marinade time: 4h00 or more

Ingredients:
16 chicken drumsticks

Tandoori mix:
250 ml (1 cup) coconut milk
Juice of 2 lemons
125 ml (½ cup) olive oil
60ml (¼ cup) tandoori spices
15 ml (1 tablespoon) red sweet paprika
Sea salt & fresh ground pepper to taste

Mango Chutney:
30 ml (2 tablespoons) olive oil
2 garlic cloves, minced
15 ml (1 tablespoon) minced fresh ginger
2 mango, peeled and cubed
30 ml (2 tablespoons) raw honey
60 ml (¼ cup) white vinegar
60 ml (¼ cup) water
2 cinnamon sticks
4 cloves
1-2 pinches of crushed chilies to taste
Sea salt & fresh ground pepper to taste

Instructions:
1. Put all the ingredients for the tandoori mix together in a zip lock bag or a container, place the chicken in, and let marinate for at least 4h00.
2. For the chutney, in a small frying pan, heat the oil on high, reduce heat to medium, and cook the garlic and ginger for 2 to 3 minutes. Add all the remaining ingredients, and cook covered for an additional 15 minutes on low heat. Remove the cover, and cook another 10 minutes or until you obtain a consistent chutney. Cool before serving
3. Pre-heat oven to 400°F.
4. Place the drumsticks on a lightly oiled baking sheet. Cook for 30 minutes until the chicken is well cooked.
5. Serve with the mango chutney and your favorite steamed vegetables.

Nutritional Information (per serving)
Calories: 444
Fat total: 40.1g, saturated fat: 14.7g
Carbohydrates: 13.3g, dietary fiber: 5.6 g
Sugars: 4.1g, protein: 14.2g

Stuffed Sea Bass

Serves: 4
Prep Time: 15 minutes
Cooking Time: 25 minutes

Ingredients:
4 sea bass, about 350 to 450 grams (¾ to 1 pound) each, cleaned, head removed
125 ml (½ cup) olive oil

45 ml (3 tablespoons) olive oil
225 g (½ pound) white mushrooms, sliced
1 tablespoon fresh parsley, minced
1 green pepper, diced
Freshly squeezed lemon juice to taste
Sea salt and fresh ground pepper to taste

Instructions:
1. Pre-heat the oven at 215°C/425°F.
2. Salt and pepper the inside of the bass. Add lemon juice to taste.
3. Place each fish on a foil sheet large enough to cover the fish.
4. Melt half of the butter in a medium-size frying pan, add the shallots, and cook 2-3 minutes. Add the mushroom, pepper, and parsley. Season with salt and pepper to taste, and cook for an additional 6 minutes until vegetables are tender.
5. Stuff each fish with ¼ of the vegetable mix, and brush the fish with olive oil. Seal the aluminum foil well. Place the foil packets on a baking sheet. Cook for 16 minutes.
6. Take out of the oven and make sure the fish is well cooked. If not, bake for an additional 2 minutes or until cooked.
7. Serve with lemon slices and your favorite vegetables.

Nutritional Information (per serving)
Calories: 444
Fat total: 40.1g, saturated fat: 14.7g
Carbohydrates: 13.3g, dietary fiber: 5.6g
Sugars: 4.1g, protein: 14.2g

Paleo Sausage Delight

Serves: 4
Prep Time: 15 minutes
Cooking Time: 25 minutes

Ingredients:
6 Paleo-approved sausages of your choice
60 ml (¼ cup) olive oil
60 ml (¼ cup) apple cider vinegar
20 white mushrooms, trimmed
¼ cup fresh flat parsley, minced
2 sweet peppers, sliced in 1-inch strips
2 red onions, sliced in ½ inch strips
Sea salt and fresh ground pepper to taste

Instructions:
1. Pre-heat the oven at 200°C/400°F.
2. In a large mixing bowl, combine all ingredients except parsley. Season with salt and freshly ground pepper to taste.
3. Lay the sausages and vegetable mix on a parchment paper-covered baking sheet, and cook for 40 minutes.
4. Sprinkle with parsley and serve with your favorite mustard and a side of slaw.

Nutritional Information (per serving)
Calories: 444
Fat total: 40.1g, Saturated fat: 14.7g
Carbohydrates: 13.3g, dietary fiber: 5.6g
Sugars: 4.1g, protein: 14.2g

Roasted Beef with Nutty Vegetables

Serves: 4
Prep Time: 15 minutes
Cooking Time: 35 minutes

Ingredients:
30 ml (2 tablespoons) olive oil
450 g (2 pounds) lean beef steak (brisket), sliced
30 ml (2 tablespoons) grainy Dijon Mustard
Montreal steak spice to taste
Garlic powder to taste
1 onion, sliced
15 ml (1 tablespoon) garlic, minced
250 ml (1 cup) asparagus, sliced
2 zucchinis, cubed
30 ml (2 tablespoons) almond butter
30 ml (2 tablespoons) almond slivers (optional)
Salt and pepper to taste

Directions:
1. Preheat the oven to 160°C/325°F.
2. Heat oil in a skillet on high heat.
3. Rub each steak with mustard, Montreal steak spices, and garlic. When the skillet is hot, stir in the steak slices, and cook for 1-2 minutes on each side until beef is nicely colored.
4. Transfer beef to a baking dish, season with salt and pepper. Place in preheated oven and bake for 10-15 minutes, depending on steak thickness and how you like your steak cooked. When the steaks are cooked to your liking, remove from oven and let rest for a few minutes before serving. This will make your steak juicier.
5. While steaks are baking, in the same skillet, add some more olive oil if necessary, sauté onions and almond

slivers (optional) for 2-3 minutes, stirring often. Add asparagus and zucchini and cook 4-5 minutes until vegetables are tender but still crispy. Remove from heat, add almond butter and parsley. Reserve.

6. Serve each steak with a generous portion of the nutty vegetables.

Nutritional Information (per serving)
Calories: 449
Fat total: 29.0g, saturated fat: 7.8g
Carbohydrates: 9.5g, Dietary fiber: 2.5g
Sugars: 3.9g, protein: 37.5g

Tilapia with Thai Curry

Serves: 2
Prep Time: 10 minutes
Cooking Time: 25 minutes

Ingredients
125 ml (½ cup) coconut milk
250 ml (1 cup) fresh basil leaves
60 ml (4 tablespoons) Thai curry paste
30 ml (2 tablespoons) olive oil
2 tilapia fillets
1 large red bell peppers, deseeded, julienne
1 onion, sliced
60 ml (¼ cup) scallions, sliced
30 ml (2 tablespoons) fish sauce*
Salt and freshly ground black pepper to taste

Directions
1. Place coconut milk, basil leaves, and Thai curry paste into a food processor and blend until smooth.
2. Heat oil in a large pan. Add tilapia fillets, and cook for 5 minutes on each side until little browned. Remove tilapia to a plate, and set aside.
3. Add red bell peppers, onion, and scallions in the same pan, and cook until the vegetables are tender.
4. Add coconut milk mixture, and cook for 5 minutes until thickens. Add in reserved fish fillets; simmer until tilapia is heated through.
5. Drizzle fish sauce, season with salt and pepper and serve.

* Make sure that the fish sauce is completely paleo, containing fish and salt only. It is suggested to read the label before purchasing.

Nutritional Information (per serving)
Calories: 441
Fat total: 29.7g, saturated fat: 15.1g
Carbohydrates: 21.1g, dietary fiber: 4.7g
Sugars: 10.6g, protein: 25.3g

Paleo Orange Chicken

Serves: 2
Prep Time: 5 minutes
Cooking Time: 20 minutes

Ingredients:
15 ml (1 tablespoon) coconut oil
225 g (½ pound) boneless chicken breast, cut into strips

1 garlic clove, minced
125 ml (½ cup) fresh orange juice
30 ml (2 tablespoons) grated orange
Salt and pepper for seasoning

Directions:
1. Heat oil in a large frying pan over medium heat.
2. Stir in garlic and sauté 1 minute. Add chicken strips, and cook a few minutes, stirring occasionally until chicken is not pink anymore.
3. Add orange juice, cover, and continue to cook for 15 minutes over medium-low, until chicken is tender and juices almost run clear.
4. Sprinkle grated orange, season with salt and pepper, and serve.

Nutritional Information (per serving)
Calories: 310
Fat total: 15.3g, saturated fat: 8.2g
Carbohydrates: 8.3g, dietary fiber: 0.0g
Sugars: 6.3g, protein: 33.5g

Beef Goulash

Serves: 4
Prep Time: 20 minutes
Cooking Time: 2h00

Ingredients:
1 kg (2 pounds) boneless stew beef such as chuck roast
30 ml (2 tablespoons) olive oil
1 large onion, chopped

4 garlic clove, minced
5 ml (1 teaspoon) caraway seeds
1 red bell pepper, deseeded, julienne
2 sweet potatoes, peeled and cubed
2 tomatoes, chopped
5 ml (1 teaspoon) salt
15 ml (1 tablespoon) jalapeños pepper, minced
500 ml (2 cups) beef broth
Salt and pepper

Directions:

1. Cut beef into same size cube, about 4-5 cm (1-2 inches). Dry beef with paper towels.
2. Heat oil in a large and deep skillet. Add beef, and brown the meat very well, in batches if necessary. For proper browning, the beef cubes should not touch each other in the pan. Remove the meat from the skillet and reserve.
3. Add oil if necessary. Sauté onions for few minutes until translucent. Add in garlic, and cook for 2 minutes. Add the spices, mix well. Add red bell peppers and tomatoes and cook for 5 minutes. Add the reserved beef
6. Season with salt and pepper to taste, and add the jalapeños chili.
7. Add broth, and bring to a boil on high heat. Reduce heat to medium-low. Cover and cook for 1h00. Add sweet potatoes, and cook for an additional 30 minutes. The meat should be very tender and easily cut with a fork. Taste and adjust seasoning with salt or pepper.
8. Serve hot with a side green salad.

Nutritional Information (per serving)
Calories: 269
Fat total: 23.7g, saturated fat: 7.5g
Carbohydrates: 6.6g, dietary fiber: 1.6g
Sugars: 3.3g, protein: 7.9g

Baked Beef with Vegetables

Serves: 4
Prep Time: 10 minutes
Marinating Time: 2 hours
Cooking Time: 35 minutes

Ingredients:
30 ml (2 tablespoons) coconut oil
225 g (½ pound) boneless beef strips
1 small red onion, chopped
2 cloves garlic, chopped
125 ml (½ cup) carrots, sliced
1000 ml (4 cups) butternut squash, chopped
1 sweet potato, chopped
2.5 ml (½ teaspoon) dried thyme
2.5 ml (½ teaspoon) dried rosemary
60 ml (¼ cup) coconut amino
2.5 ml (½ teaspoon) ground black pepper

Directions:
1. In a large bowl, add all ingredients except vegetables. Mix well. Let marinate for 30 minutes.
2. Preheat the oven to 180ºC/350° F.
3. Toss in vegetables as well.
4. Place beef and vegetables in the baking dish, cover the dish completely with foil, and bake for 30 to 35 minutes. After that, remove foil, and roast again for 10 minutes.

Nutritional Information (per serving)
Calories: 353
Fat total: 27.6g, saturated fat: 14.9g
Carbohydrates: 17.8g, dietary fiber: 3.3g
Sugars: 4.8g, protein: 9.8g

Herb-Crusted Pork Tenderloin

Serves: 4
Prep Time: 15 minutes
Marinating Time: 2 hours
Cooking Time: 40 minutes

Ingredients:
2 pork tenderloins, about 350 to 450 g (¾ to 1 pound) each
2 cloves garlic, minced
45 ml (3 tablespoons) fresh rosemary
45 ml (3 tablespoons) fresh thyme
15 ml (1 tablespoon) smoked paprika
½ onion, cut in a few pieces
5 ml (1 teaspoon) sea salt
5 ml (1 teaspoon) ground black pepper
60 ml (¼ cup) freshly squeezed lime juice

Directions:
1. Preheat the oven to 180°C/350°F.
2. In a food processor, add all ingredients except pork. Pulse until it becomes a smooth paste.
3. In a bowl, add pork and herb mixture. Mix until well combined. Cover and refrigerate for 2 hours to marinate.
4. Place pork into baking dish. Bake for 30 to 40 minutes until pork is fully cooked.
5. Cut into slices before serving.
6. Serve with a medley of steamed vegetables and unsweetened organic applesauce if desired.

Nutritional Information (per serving)
Calories: 165
Fat total: 5.9g, saturated fat: 2.3g
Carbohydrates: 9.4g, dietary fiber: 2.9g
Sugars: 1.1g, protein: 20.3g

Pork Chops with Apple

Serves: 2
Prep Time: 10 minutes
Cooking Time: 20 minutes

Ingredients:
15 ml (1 tablespoon) coconut oil
2 pork chops
1 large onion, sliced
2 apples, sliced
Salt and freshly ground black pepper to taste

Directions:
1. Heat oil in a large pan.
2. Put chops in the pan, and cook for 5 minutes on each side until golden browned.
3. Add onion and apples, and continue to cook for 7 to 9 minutes until the onion and apples are tender.
4. Sprinkle with salt and pepper and serve.

Nutritional Information (per serving)
Calories: 439
Fat total: 26.7g, saturated fat: 13.3g
Carbohydrates: 31.9g, dietary fiber: 5.9g
 Sugars: 21.9g, protein: 18.7g

Ground Beef with Kale

Serves: 2
Prep Time: 10 minutes
Cooking Time: 15minutes

Ingredients:
15 ml (1 tablespoon) coconut oil
225 g (½ pound) ground beef
2 small red chilies, finely sliced
1 large bunch of kale, trimmed and chopped
1 lemon
Salt and pepper for seasoning

Directions:
1. Heat oil in a large frying pan.
2. Stir in beef and red chilies, cook for few minutes until little browned.
3. Add kale, and continue to cook until the kale is just wilted.
4. Drizzle lemon juice, season with salt and pepper and serve.

Nutritional Information (per serving)
Calories: 295
Fat total: 14.2g, saturated fat: 8.7g
Carbohydrates: 4.7g, dietary fiber: 0.7g.
Sugars: 0.0g, protein: 35.9g

Seasoned Slow Cooker Turkey Breast

Serves: 6-8
Prep Time: 10 minutes
Cooking Time: 8 hours

Ingredients:
1 large turkey breast roast (1½ to 2 kg /3 to 4 pounds)
1 onion, cut into 3 large slices of equal thickness
5 garlic cloves, minced or 15 ml (3 teaspoons) garlic powder
45 ml (3 tablespoons) raw honey
60 ml (¼ cup) coconut amino
30 ml (2 tablespoons) melted duck fat or olive oil
30 ml (2 tablespoons) smoked paprika
15 ml (1 tablespoon) dry thyme
5 ml (1 teaspoon) pepper

Directions:
1. Preheat the slow cooker at low heat.
2. Place the onion slices in the bottom of the slow cooker, and set the turkey on them.
3. In a small mixing bowl, combine paprika, garlic, thyme, raw honey, coconut amino, melted duck fat (or olive oil). Brush the turkey breast with the spice mix. Season with salt and pepper to taste.
4. Set the slow cooker or a timer for 5h30. The internal temperature of the turkey should read 75ºC/165ºF
5. Serve with mashed sweet potatoes and steamed in-season vegetables.

Note: If you don't have a slow cooker, you can use a Dutch oven and bake the turkey for 5h00-6h00 in the oven at 140ºC/275 F, or until the turkey is cooked throughout.

Nutritional Information (per serving)
Calories: 566
Fat total: 20.0g, saturated fat: 6.0g
Carbohydrates: 20.0g, dietary fiber: 1.4g
Sugars: 17.8g, protein: 85.0g

Marinated Grilled Spicy Beef

Serves: 2
Prep Time: 10 minutes
Marinating time: 2h00
Cooking Time: 10 minutes

Ingredients:
2 -175 g (6 oz.) sirloin steaks
30 ml (2 tablespoons) olive oil
30 ml (2 tablespoons) lemon juice
1 clove garlic, finely chopped
1 ml (¼ teaspoon) cayenne pepper
5 ml (1 teaspoon) chili powder
5 ml (1 teaspoon) green chili, chopped
2.5 ml (½ teaspoon) oregano
1 ml (¼ teaspoon) salt
2.5 ml (½ teaspoon) freshly ground black pepper

Directions:
1. Combine all ingredients in a bowl and mix together.
2. Leave marinated for at least 2 hours.
3. Preheat a grill pan to high.
4. Place steaks on a grill pan over high heat.
5. Grill for 3 minutes on each side for a medium-cooked steak, or until to your desired doneness.

Nutritional Information (per serving)
Calories: 375
Fat total: 21.0g, saturated fat: 5.2g
Carbohydrates: 3.4g, dietary fiber: 1.2g
Sugars: 0.7g, protein: 13.6g

Sautéed Juicy Pork Tenderloin with Peaches

Serves: 2
Prep Time: 10 minutes
Cooking Time: 35-40 minutes

Ingredients:
15 ml (1 tablespoon) coconut oil
1 onion, chopped
225 g (½ pound) pork tenderloin, sliced
2 peaches, sliced (you can also use frozen peaches)
30 ml (2 tablespoons) rosemary
250 ml (1 cup) beef broth
30 ml (2 tablespoons) apple cider vinegar
Salt and pepper to taste

Directions:
1. Heat oil in a large saucepan over medium.
2. Stir in onion and sauté until onion is translucent. Add pork and cook for few minutes until pork is a little browned.
3. Add peaches, rosemary, and beef broth, cover and continue to cook for 30 minutes until the pork is tender and gravy thickens a little.
4. Drizzle vinegar, season with salt and pepper and serve.

Nutritional Information (per serving)
Calories: 324
Fat total: 12.0g, saturated fat: 7.7g
Carbohydrates: 20.3g, dietary fiber: 4.7g
Sugars: 12.1g, protein: 32.8g

Hearty Beef and Vegetable Stew

Serves: 2
Prep Time: 10 minutes
Cooking Time: 50 minutes

Ingredients:
30 ml (2 tablespoons) olive oil
1 onion, sliced
225 g (½ pound) boneless beef (chuck roast)
1 carrot, cubed
1 potato, cubed
2.5 ml (½ teaspoon) rosemary, chopped
125 ml (½ cup) tomato paste
Salt and pepper to taste
1 ml (¼ teaspoon) raw honey

Directions:
1. Heat oil in a large stew pot.
2. Stir in onion and beef stew, cook for 5 minutes until beef is tender.
3. Add carrots, potato, rosemary, and tomato paste and cook for 5 minutes.
4. Season with salt and pepper.
5. Add broth, bring to a boil, cover, and cook on medium heat for 40 minutes.

6. Drizzle with honey and serve.

Nutritional Information (per serving)
Calories: 418
Fat total: 19.5g, saturated fat: 4.1g
Carbohydrates: 36.1g, dietary fiber: 6.7g
Sugars: 13.0g, protein: 29.5g

Butterfish with Lemongrass

Serves: 2
Prep Time: 10 minutes
Cooking Time: 15 minutes

Ingredients:
30 ml (2 tablespoons) olive oil
2 butterfish fillets
15 ml (1 tablespoon) fresh lemongrass, chopped
1 jalapeño, chopped
1 ml (¼ teaspoon) raw honey

Directions:
1. Heat oil in a large frying pan.
2. Add in butterfish fillets, and cook for 8 to 10 minutes until fillets are cooked.
3. Add lemongrass and jalapeño, and cook for 5 minutes. Season with salt.
4. Drizzle fish with honey and serve.

Nutritional Information (per serving)
Calories: 347
Fat total: 25.9g, saturated fat: 8.4g
Carbohydrates: 6.0g, dietary fiber: 0.0g
Sugars: 3.8g, protein: 23.8g

Baked Chicken with Olives

Serves: 4
Prep Time: 10 minutes
Cooking Time: 20 minutes

Ingredients:
4 chicken thighs (4 ounces each)
125 ml (½ cup) olives, sliced
60 ml (4 tablespoons) raw honey
2 garlic cloves
5 ml (1 teaspoon) fresh lemon juice
4 teaspoon coconut oil

Directions:
1. Preheat the oven to 180ºC/350°F. Lightly grease a baking dish.
2. Combine all ingredients in a bowl and mix well.
3. Put chicken mixture over the baking dish.
4. Bake for 15-20 minutes, or until chicken thighs are cooked through.

Nutritional Information (per serving)
Calories: 340, fat total: 14.7g, saturated fat: 6.5g
Carbohydrates: 18.9g, dietary fiber: 0.6g
Sugars: 17.3g, protein: 33.1g

Primal Chicken Fajitas

Serves: 2
Prep Time: 10 minutes
Cooking Time: 10 minutes

Ingredients:
1 skinless and boneless chicken breast cut in strips
1 medium onion, thickly sliced
½ red bell pepper, deseeded, julienne
½ green bell pepper, deseeded, julienne
1 tomato, deseeded, sliced
2.5 ml (½ teaspoon) chili powder
2.5 ml (½ teaspoon) cumin
2.5 ml (½ teaspoon) coriander
2.5 ml (½ teaspoon) oregano
5 ml (1 teaspoon) lemon juice
Pinch of salt and freshly ground black pepper
30 ml (2 tablespoons) olive oil

Directions:
1. Toss chicken and vegetables in a bowl with oil and sprinkle with salt and pepper.
2. Heat oil in a large skillet.
3. Stir in onion and chicken, and cook for 10 minutes or until chicken is almost done.
4. Now, add in vegetables, sprinkle with herbs and spices. Cook for 5 minutes until vegetables are crisply tender. Lastly, drizzle with lemon juice and serve.

Note you can add avocados, pickles, and salsa as well.*

Nutritional Information (per serving)
Calories: 232
Fat total: 16.0g, saturated fat: 2.3g
Carbohydrates: 10.6g, dietary fiber: 3.2g
Sugars: 5.6g, protein: 13.6g

Liver with Onions

Serves: 2
Prep Time: 5 minutes
Cooking Time: 15 minutes

Ingredients:
30 ml (2 tablespoons) olive oil
2 medium onions, thickly sliced
2 slices of beef liver, strips
2.5 ml (½ teaspoon) oregano
5 ml (1 teaspoon) lemon juice
Salt and freshly ground black pepper

Directions:
1. Heat 15 ml (1 tablespoon) olive oil in a frying pan.
2. Stir in onion and cook until onions are tender and caramelized, about 5 minutes.
3. Remove from pan and set aside.
4. Heat remaining 15 ml (1 tablespoon) olive oil in the same frying pan.
5. Add beef liver, and cook for 3 minutes on each side until tender.
6. Sprinkle with oregano, lemon juice, season with salt and pepper.
7. Serve liver with caramelized onions.

Nutritional Information (per serving)
Calories: 455
Fat total: 18.6g, saturated fat: 4.3g
Carbohydrates: 16.9g, dietary fiber: 1.6g
Sugars: 3.0g, protein: 52.9g

Roasted Salmon with Bacon

Serves: 4
Prep Time: 10 minutes
Cooking Time: 25minutes

Ingredients:
250 ml (1 cup) almond flour
250 ml (1 cup) coconut flour
Salt and black pepper for seasoning
450 g (1 pound) salmon fillets
2 eggs, beaten
60 ml (4 tablespoons) almond butter, melted
4 slices paleo-approved bacon
15 ml (1 tablespoon) coconut oil

Directions:
1. Preheat the oven to 200°C/400°F. Lightly grease a baking dish.
2. Mix almond flour, coconut flour, salt, and black pepper in a bowl.
3. In another bowl, whisk the eggs.
4. Dip fish fillets in the eggs then into the flour mixture. Set aside.

5. Put bacon slices in a bowl, add coconut oil, and season with salt and pepper.
6. Put fish fillets in the baking dish with bacon slices, brush with melted almond butter, and bake for 20-25 minutes.

Nutritional Information (per serving)
Calories: 611
Fat total: 38.2g, saturated fat: 10.0g
Carbohydrates: 20.9g, dietary fiber: 11.3g
Sugars: 2.6g, protein: 43.5g

Curried Pork Chops

Serves: 2
Prep Time: 5 minutes
Cooking Time: 35 minutes

Ingredients:
15 ml (1 tablespoon) coconut oil
1 clove garlic, minced
5 ml (1 teaspoon) ginger, chopped
225 g (½ pound) boneless lean pork loin chops
5 ml (1 teaspoon) chili powder
15 ml (1 tablespoon) curry powder
5 ml (1 teaspoon) paprika
125 ml (½ cup) coconut milk
2.5 ml (½ teaspoon) salt
2.5 ml (½ teaspoon) ground black pepper

Directions:
1. Heat oil in a pan on medium-high.
2. Stir in garlic and ginger, cook for few minutes until ginger and garlic are tender and fragrant.
3. Add chops, and cook for 5 minutes on each side until lightly browned.
4. Add chili powder, curry powder, paprika, and milk. Bring to a boil on high heat.
5. Season with salt and pepper. Cover and cook on medium low heat for 20 to 25 minutes, or until pork is cooked through.

Nutritional Information (per serving)
Calories: 320
Fat total: 25.0g, saturated fat: 20.2g
Carbohydrates: 7.6g, dietary fiber: 3.3g
Sugars: 2.3g, protein: 20.3g

Spicy Mixed Vegetable Curry

Serves: 2
Prep Time: 20 minutes
Cooking Time: 30 minutes

Ingredients:
15 ml (1 tablespoon) coconut oil
1 onion, chopped
3 clove garlic, minced
5 ml (1 teaspoon) fresh ginger, grated
60 ml (¼ cup) carrots, cubed
60 ml (¼ cup) broccoli, cubed
60 ml (¼ cup) zucchini, cube

60 ml (¼ cup) mushrooms
125 ml (½ cup) coconut milk
5 ml (1 teaspoon) ground cumin
2.5 ml (½ teaspoon) ground coriander
2.5 ml (½ teaspoon) ground turmeric
1 ml (¼ teaspoon) cayenne pepper
1 ml (¼ teaspoon) ground nutmeg
Salt and pepper for seasoning

Directions:
1. Warm oil in a large frying pan on medium-high heat.
2. Stir in onion, garlic, and ginger and cook for a few minutes until onion is translucent.
3. Add carrots, broccoli, zucchini, and mushrooms and continue to cook for 10 minutes until vegetables are crisply tender.
4. Add coconut milk, sprinkle cumin, coriander, turmeric, cayenne pepper, and nutmeg. Season with salt and pepper, and cook for 5 to 8 minutes until the gravy thickens.
5. Serve hot sprinkled with freshly chopped coriander.

Nutritional Information (per serving)
Calories: 250
Fat total: 21.7g, saturated fat: 18.7g
Carbohydrates: 14.3g, dietary fiber: 3.9g
Sugars: 5.6g, protein: 3.5g

Fish Curry with Bananas

Serves: 2
Prep Time: 10 minutes
Cooking Time: 20 minutes

Ingredients:
30 ml (2 tablespoons) olive oil
1 onion, sliced
2 tilapia fillets, strips
125 ml (½ cup) coconut milk
½ tablespoon red curry paste
5 ml (1 teaspoon) lemon juice
1 banana, sliced
15 ml (1 tablespoon) almonds, chopped
125 ml (½ cup) fresh cilantro, chopped
1 lemon, sliced
Pinch of salt and freshly ground black pepper

Directions:
1. Warm oil in a large frying pan on medium heat.
2. Stir in onion and tilapia fillets, cook for 8 to 10 minutes until tilapia is cooked.
3. Add coconut milk, red curry paste, and lemon juice and cook for 2 minutes.
4. Add banana slices and almonds, and cook for 5 minutes. season with salt and pepper
5. Sprinkle with cilantro and lemon slices and serve.

Nutritional Information (per serving)
Calories: 312
Fat total: 21.5g, Saturated fat: 10.5g
Carbohydrates: 17.4g, dietary fiber: 3.5g
Sugars: 8.2g, protein: 16.4g

Honey Mustard Beef

Serves: 2
Prep Time: 5 minutes
Cooking Time: 35 minutes

Ingredients:
225 g (½ pound) top sirloin beef, cut into strips
2.5 ml (½ teaspoon) sea salt
2.5 ml (½ teaspoon) ground black pepper
30 ml (2 tablespoons) raw honey
30 ml (2 tablespoons) ground mustard
125 ml (½ cup) beef broth

Directions:
1. Preheat the oven to 180ºC/350°F.
2. In a large bowl, add all ingredients and mix well.
3. Put beef in the baking dish, and bake for 30 to 35 minutes.
4. Serve in a platter along with your favorite steamed vegetables.

Nutritional Information (per serving)
Calories: 318
Fat total: 12.6g, saturated fat: 4.3g,
Carbohydrates: 21.8g, dietary fiber: 1.8g
Sugars: 18.2g, protein: 28.2g

DESSERTS RECIPES
Quick Chocolate Bonbon

Serves: 4-6
Prep Time: 20 minutes
Cooking Time: 5-10 minutes
Freezing Time: 20 minutes

Ingredients:
125 ml (½ cup) dark chocolate chunks (70% or more cocoa)
250 ml (1 cup) raspberry, packed (fresh or frozen)
15 ml (1 tablespoon) of raw honey
5 ml (1 teaspoon) crushed almonds

Directions:
1. Melt chocolate over double boiler. You can also microwave the chocolate until just melted.
2. Take a paintbrush, and brush a mini cupcake mold or a candy mold with the chocolate. Paint thickly all around walls and base of the cups, remembering to keep some melted chocolate for covering the candies.
3. Place in freezer to set for 10 minutes.
4. In the meantime, puree the raspberry in a blender or food processor until smooth, and strain it through a fine sieve to remove the seeds. Add the raw honey to the raspberry puree, and mix well. Set aside
5. After 10 minutes, remove from freezer. Equally, spoon the raspberry puree in all the chocolate molds. Sprinkle with crushed almonds. Paint the top with the melted chocolate to cover the bonbons.
6. Place in freezer again to harden for 10 minutes.
7. Lastly, pop the candies out of the mold into a plate, keeping upside down and serve.

This recipe makes around 18 bonbons depending on mold size.

Nutritional Information (per serving)
Calories: 238
Fat total: 13.0g, saturated fat: 8.8g
Carbohydrates: 27.1g, dietary fiber: 2.1g
Sugars: 22.7g, protein: 3.6g

Ginger Brownies

Serves: 2
Prep Time: 5 minutes
Cooking Time: 25 minutes

Ingredients:
500 ml (2 cups) almond flour
125 ml (½ cup) coconut flour
60 ml (4 tablespoons) cocoa powder, unsweetened
0.5 ml (⅛ teaspoon) cinnamon
Pinch of salt
2 eggs
30 ml (2 tablespoons) coconut oil
30 ml (2 tablespoons) raw honey
15 ml (1 teaspoon) pure vanilla extract
1 teaspoon ground nutmeg
1 ml (¼ teaspoon) fresh ginger, minced

Directions:
1. Preheat the oven to 200°C/400°F. Lightly grease a baking pan.
2. Mix almond flour, coconut flour, cocoa powder, cinnamon, and salt in a bowl.

3. In another, bowl whisk the eggs.
4. Mix eggs with flour mixture and remaining ingredients.
5. Place into the baking pan.
6. Bake for 20-25 minutes until a toothpick inserted in the center comes out clean.

Nutritional Information (per serving)
Calories: 269
Fat total: 21.1g, saturated fat: 9.7g
Carbohydrates: 20.2g, dietary fiber: 4.4
Sugars: 12.7g, protein: 7.2g

Cherry and Almond Butter Milkshake

Serves: 2
Prep Time: 5 minutes
Cooking Time: 0 minutes

Ingredients:
1cup almond milk
1 whole banana, frozen
8 cherries, frozen
30 ml (2 tablespoons) almond butter
15 ml (1 tablespoon) honey
Ice cubes, as many as you like

Directions:
1. Place all the ingredients into a food processor, and blend until smooth and creamy. Serve and enjoy!

Nutritional Information (per serving)
Calories: 336
Fat total: 25.2g, saturated fat: 17.5g
Carbohydrates: 28.0g, dietary fiber: 3.3g
Sugars: 13.2g, protein: 4.6g

Banana with Coconut & Almond Butter

Serves: 2
Prep Time: 10 minutes
Cooking Time: 0 minutes

Ingredients:
2 bananas, sliced
60 ml (4 tablespoons) coconut milk
60 ml (4 tablespoons) almond butter
0.5 ml (⅛ teaspoon) cinnamon

Directions:
1. Toss all ingredients in a mixing bowl, and sprinkle with cinnamon. Let it rest 5 minutes before serving in dessert bowls.

Nutritional Information (per serving)
Calories: 378
Fat total: 25.6g, saturated fat: 8.1g
Carbohydrates: 34.4g, dietary fiber: 5.0g
Sugars: 15.4g, protein: 8.8g

Paleo Pumpkin Muffins

Serves: 5
Prep Time: 2 minutes
Cooking Time: 25 minutes

Ingredients:
750 ml (1½ cup) almond flour
60 ml (4 tablespoons) coconut flour
5 ml (1 teaspoon) baking soda
5 ml (1 teaspoon) baking powder
2.5 ml (½ teaspoon) pumpkin pie spice
2.5 ml (½ teaspoon) ground cinnamon
0.5 ml (⅛ teaspoon) sea salt
2 large eggs
¾ cup pumpkin puree
60 ml (¼ cup) raw honey
30 ml (2 teaspoons) almond butter
15 ml (1 tablespoon) almonds, toasted and chopped

Directions:
1. Preheat the oven to 200°C/400°F.
2. Whisk almond flour, coconut flour, baking soda, baking powder, and pumpkin pie spice in a mixing bowl. Sprinkle with cinnamon and salt.
3. In another bowl whisk the eggs. Add pumpkin puree, honey, and butter.
4. Mix wet ingredients with dry ingredients. Fill the batter in muffin cups until each is almost full.
5. Sprinkle with almonds.
6. Bake for 20 to 25 minutes, or until a toothpick inserted in the center comes out clean.

Nutritional Information (per serving)
Calories: 189
Fat total: 8.7g, saturated fat: 1.4g
Carbohydrates: 23.7, dietary fiber: 4.5g
Sugars: 16.1g, protein: 6.3g

Coconut Whipped Cream

Serves: 2
Prep Time: 5 minutes
Refrigerating Time: 2-3 hours

Ingredients:
250 ml (1 cup) coconut cream
250 ml (1 cup) coconut milk
1 ml (¼ teaspoon) cinnamon
2.5 ml (½ teaspoon) vanilla extract
1 ml (¼ teaspoon) ground nutmeg

Directions:
1. Place all the ingredients in food processor, and blend until smooth and creamy.
2. Pour coconut cream in 4 cups, and refrigerate for at least 2 to 3 hours.
3. Serve and enjoy!

Nutritional Information (per serving)
Calories: 559
Fat total: 57.6g, saturated fat: 51.0g
Carbohydrates: 14.0g, dietary fiber: 5.6g
Sugars: 8.4g, protein: 5.6g

Creamy Banana Treat with Cranberries and Coconut

Serves: 2
Prep Time: 5 minutes
Cooking Time: 0 minutes

Ingredients:
1 large banana, sliced
30 ml (2 tablespoons) almond butter
30 ml (2 tablespoons) coconut milk
125 ml (½ cup) cranberries
Pinch of cinnamon

Directions:
1. Combine bananas with almond butter and coconut milk in a large bowl.
2. Add cranberries on top and sprinkle with cinnamon before serving.

Nutritional Information (per serving)
Calories: 208
Fat total: 12.9g, saturated fat: 4.1g
Carbohydrates: 22.2g, dietary fiber: 3.9g
Sugars: 9.8g, protein: 4.6g,

Berries with Almonds

Serves: 2
Prep Time: 5 minutes
Cooking Time: 0minutes

Ingredients:
250 ml (1 cup) fresh berries
30 ml (2 tablespoons) balsamic vinegar
30 ml (2 tablespoons) maple syrup
85 ml (⅓ cup) almonds, toasted, and chopped

Directions:
1. Combine all ingredients in a bowl and serve.

Nutritional Information (per serving)
Calories: 181
Fat total: 8.1g, saturated fat: 0.6g
Carbohydrates: 25.5g, Dietary fiber: 4.5g
Sugars: 17.6g, protein: 3.8g

Sweet & Salty Chocolate Barks

Serves: 4
Prep Time: 5 minutes
Cooking Time: 3 minute
Refrigerating Time: 1 hour

Ingredients:
125 ml (½ cup) dark chocolate (70% or more cocoa), chopped
125 ml (½ cup) dried cherries, chopped
250 ml (1 cup) pecans

1 ml (¼ teaspoon) fleur de sel or any coarse salt

Directions:
1. Melt chocolate in a double boiler saucepan on medium-low heat, or in the microwave until just melted.
2. Stir in cherries, pecans, and salt, and cook for few seconds.
3. Spread chocolate mixture on a baking dish with a spatula.
4. Refrigerate for at least 1 hour until set.
5. Break into bite-size pieces, serve, and enjoy!

Nutritional Information (per serving)
Calories: 221
Fat total: 16.0g, saturated fat: 5.2g
Carbohydrates: 18.1g, dietary fiber: 2.1g
Sugars: 11.4g, protein: 2.9g

Honey Coated Walnuts & Peaches

Serves: 2
Prep Time: 5 minutes
Cooking Time: 3minutes

Ingredients:
30 ml (2 tablespoons) almond butter
60 ml (4 tablespoons) raw honey
2 peaches, sliced
60 ml (4 tablespoons) walnuts, chopped
5 ml (1 teaspoon) ground cinnamon

Directions:
1. Heat butter and honey in a saucepan.
2. Stir in peach and walnuts and cook for 3 minutes.
3. Sprinkle with cinnamon. Serve and enjoy!

Nutritional Information (per serving)
Calories: 367
Fat total: 18.5g, saturated fat: 1.4g
Carbohydrates: 49.3g, dietary fiber: 3.8g
Sugars: 42.9g, protein: 8.2g

Almond Florentine

Serves: 2
Prep Time: 10 minutes
Cooking Time: 30 minutes

Ingredients:
125 ml (½ cup) almond meal
2.5 ml (½ teaspoon) cinnamon
30 ml (2 tablespoons) nutmeg
2.5 ml (½ teaspoon) vanilla extract
45 ml (3 tablespoons) maple syrup
Pinch of salt

Directions:
1. Preheat the oven to 180°C/350°F. Lightly grease a baking dish.
2. Combine all ingredients in a bowl, and mix well.
3. Put small portions of the dough with a spoon on the baking dish.
4. Bake for 25 to 30 minutes.

Nutritional Information (per serving)
Calories: 256,
Fat total: 14.3g, saturated fat: 2.7g
Carbohydrates: 29.3g, dietary fiber: 4.7g
Sugars: 20.9g, protein: 5.5g

Apple Pudding with Coconut Whipped Cream

Serves: 2
Prep Time: 5 minutes
Cooking Time: 5 minutes

Ingredients:
45 ml (3 tablespoons) coconut oil
250 ml (1 cup) coconut milk
30 ml (2 tablespoons) raw honey
2 apples, peeled and sliced
5 ml (1 teaspoon) cinnamon
125 ml (½ cup) coconut cream
5 ml (1 teaspoon) vanilla

Directions:
1. Heat oil in a large pan.
2. Add coconut milk, honey, and apples. Cook for 5 minutes until apples are tender. Remove from the heat. Let it cool.
3. Place apple mixture in a food processor, and pulse until smooth.
4. In a small mixing bowl, add coconut cream and vanilla. With an electric mixer, whip the cream until it forms peaks and has a whipped cream texture, about 3 minutes. Add raw honey, and mix in with a spoon

5. Sprinkle with cinnamon, and serve with the coconut whipped cream.

Nutritional Information (per serving)
Calories: 319
Fat total: 12.1 g, saturated fat: 10.9
Carbohydrates: 54.5, dietary fiber: 5.0g
Sugars: 28.6g, protein: 1.5g

Raspberry Ice Cream

Serves: 2
Prep Time: 10 minutes
Cooking Time: 0 minutes

Ingredients:
250 ml (1 cup) coconut milk
60 ml (¼ cup) raw honey
125 ml (½ cup) raspberry, pureed
5 ml (1 teaspoon) vanilla extract
2.5 ml (½ teaspoon) pumpkin pie spice

For garnishing
30 ml (2 tablespoons) walnuts, chopped

Directions:
1. In a bowl, add all ice cream ingredients, and mix till well combined. Pour into ice cream maker.
2. Freeze ice cream until fully set.
3.   Garnish with walnuts.

Chocolate Pudding

Serves: 2
Prep Time: 3 minutes
Refrigerating Time: 1 hour
Cooking Time: 0 minutes

Ingredients:
30 ml (2 tablespoons) cocoa powder
1 avocado, chopped
125 ml (½ cup) almond milk
60 ml (4 tablespoons) raw honey
5 ml (1 teaspoon) vanilla extract

Directions:
1. Place all the ingredients into a food processor, and blend until smooth and creamy.
2. Refrigerate for 1 hour until set.
3. Serve chilled and enjoy!

Nutritional Information (per serving)
Calories: 320,
Fat total: 23.1g, saturated fat: 10.2g
Carbohydrates: 27.8g, dietary fiber: 6.5g
Sugars: 25.0g, protein: 2.9g

Crunchy Baked Apples

Serves: 2
Prep Time: 15 minutes
Cooking Time: 45minutes

Ingredients:
2 red apples, cored (but not peeled)
30 ml (2 tablespoons) almond butter
30 ml (2 teaspoons) cinnamon
30 ml (2 tablespoons) nutmeg
30 ml (2 tablespoons) maple syrup
30 ml (2 tablespoons) walnuts, chopped

Directions:
1. Preheat the oven to 180°C/350°F. Lightly grease a baking dish.
2. Add almond butter into apples' core cavity. Sprinkle with cinnamon and nutmeg.
3. Put apples in the baking dish. Bake for 35-45 minutes or until tender and caramelized.
4. Place the walnuts on top of each apple and drizzle with maple syrup. Let cool for 10-15 minutes.
5. Serve when apples are still warm.

Nutritional Information (per serving)
Calories: 340
Fat total: 16.6g, saturated fat: 3.1g
Carbohydrates: 47.7g, dietary fiber: 8.1g
Sugars: 33.1g, protein: 5.0g

Coconut Squares

Serves: 4
Prep Time: 5 minutes
Cooking Time: 30 minutes

Ingredients:
3 eggs
125 ml (½ cup) coconut milk
30 ml (2 tablespoons) coconut oil
30 ml (2 tablespoons) raw honey
5 ml (1 teaspoon) vanilla extract
125 ml (½ cup) almond flour
15 ml (1 tablespoon) coconut flour
1 125 ml (½ cup) unsweetened coconut, shredded
1 ml (¼ teaspoon) salt

Directions:
1. Preheat the oven to 180°C/350°F. Lightly grease a baking dish.
2. Place all ingredients in a food processor, and pulse until thick batter forms.
3. Pour batter in the baking dish. Bake for 30 minutes until edges are golden browned.
4. Remove from oven. Let it cool. Cut into squares and serve.

Nutritional Information (per serving)
Calories: 344
Fat total: 29.2g, saturated fat: 22.3g
Carbohydrates: 17.0g, dietary fiber: 4.4g
Sugars: 12.1g, protein: 6.9g

Baked Pears

Serves: 2
Prep Time: 5 minutes
Cooking Time: 15 minutes

Ingredients:
2 ripe pears, halved
5 ml (1 teaspoon) almond butter
30 m (2 teaspoons) raw honey
5 ml (1 teaspoon) fresh lemon juice
1 ml (¼ teaspoon) ground cinnamon
1 ml (¼ teaspoon) ground nutmeg

Directions:
1   Preheat the oven to 180°C/350°F. Lightly grease a baking dish.
2   Combine all ingredients in a bowl, and mix well.
3   Put pears on the baking dish.
4   Bake for 10 to 15 minutes or until the pears are done.

Nutritional Information (per serving)
Calories: 162
Fat total: 1.9g, saturated fat: 0.0g
Carbohydrates: 39.0g, dietary fiber: 6.8g,
Sugars: 26.4g, protein: 1.4g

Banana Bites

Serves: 2
Prep Time: 5 minutes
Cooking Time: 0 minutes

Ingredients:
60 ml (¼ cup) almond butter
2 bananas, sliced
15 ml (1 tablespoon) honey
5 ml (1 teaspoon) cinnamon

Directions:
1. Spread butter on banana slices.
2. Drizzle with honey and sprinkle with cinnamon.
3. Serve and enjoy!

Nutritional Information (per serving)
Calories: 338
Fat total: 18.1g, saturated fat: 1.8g
Carbohydrates: 42.1g, dietary fiber: 4.9g
Sugars: 23.0g, protein: 8.0g

Maple Paleo Bread

Serves: 4
Prep Time: 5 minutes
Cooking Time: 30 minutes

Ingredients:
250 ml (1 cup) coconut flour, sifted
2.5 ml (½ teaspoon) baking soda

2.5 ml (½ teaspoon) salt
6 eggs, lightly whisked
60 ml (4 tablespoons) maple syrup
125 ml (½ cup) coconut oil, melted

Instructions:
1. Preheat the oven to 180°C/350°F. Lightly, grease and flour a loaf pan.
2. In a bowl, mix flour, baking soda, and salt. In another bowl, whisk eggs with maple syrup and butter.
3. Add flour mixture to egg mixture, and mix till well combined.
4. Place the batter in the loaf pan. Bake for 25 to 30 minutes or until a toothpick inserted in the center comes out clean.
5. Remove from oven. Let it cool. Cut into slices and serve with coconut butter.

Nutritional Information (per serving)
Calories: 435
Fat total: 32.6g, saturated fat: 17.6g
Carbohydrates: 19.9g, dietary fiber: 10.0g
Sugars: 5.5g, protein: 12.5g

Creamy Berries

Serves: 2
Prep Time: 5 minutes
Refrigeration Time: 2 hours

Ingredients:
125 ml (½ cup) coconut milk
125 ml (½ cup) coconut cream
30 ml (2 tablespoons) strawberries
30 ml (2 tablespoons) blueberries
30 ml (2 tablespoons) blackberries
30 ml (2 tablespoons) raspberries

Directions:
1. Place all the ingredients in a food processor, and blend until smooth and creamy.
2. Place creamy berries in a bowl. Refrigerate bowl for 2 hours until set.
3. Serve and enjoy!

Nutritional Information (per serving)
Calories: 292
Fat total: 28.8g, saturated fat: 25.4g
Carbohydrates: 10.4g, dietary fiber: 4.5g
Sugars: 6.1g, protein: 3.1g

Carrot Cake Bites

Serves: 2
Prep Time: 10 minutes
Refrigerating Time: 1 hour

Ingredients:
2 medium carrots, chopped
125 ml (½ cup) raw walnuts
60 ml (¼ cup) raw cashews
85 ml (¾ cup) unsweetened dry cranberries, chopped
5 ml (1 teaspoon) grated ginger
5 ml (1 teaspoon) cinnamon
5 ml (1 teaspoon) orange zest, optional
125 ml (½ cup) organic unsweetened shredded coconut

Directions:
1. Place all the ingredients in a food processor, and pulse until a dough forms.
2. Shape the dough into small balls. Take shredded coconut in a plate. Roll balls into shredded coconut.
3. Refrigerate for 1 hour until set.
4. Serve chilled and enjoy!

Nutritional Information (per serving)
Calories: 274
Fat total: 22.2g, saturated fat: 5.7g
Carbohydrates: 15.8g, dietary fiber: 5.8g
Sugars: 4.6g, protein: 7.8g

RECIPE INDEX

DESSERTS RECIPES _____123

Also by Madison Miller

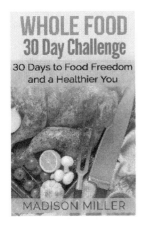
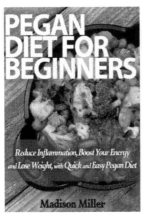
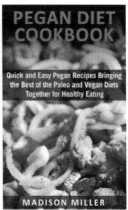

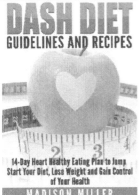
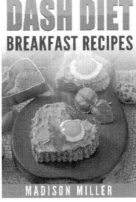
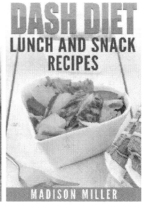

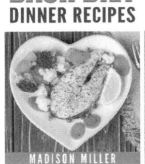
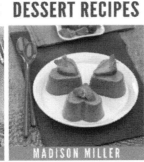
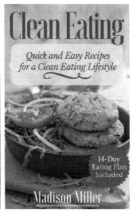

APPENDIX

Cooking Conversion Charts

1. Measuring Equivalent Chart

Type	Imperial	Imperial	Metric
Weight	1 dry ounce		28g
	1 pound	16 dry ounces	0.45 kg
Volume	1 teaspoon		5 ml
	1 dessert spoon	2 teaspoons	10 ml
	1 tablespoon	3 teaspoons	15 ml
	1 Australian tablespoon	4 teaspoons	20 ml
	1 fluid ounce	2 tablespoons	30 ml
	1 cup	16 tablespoons	240 ml
	1 cup	8 fluid ounces	240 ml
	1 pint	2 cups	470 ml
	1 quart	2 pints	0.95 l
	1 gallon	4 quarts	3.8 l
Length	1 inch		2.54 cm

* Numbers are rounded to the closest equivalent

2. Oven Temperature Equivalent Chart

Fahrenheit (°F)	Celsius (°C)	Gas Mark
220	100	
225	110	1/4
250	120	1/2
275	140	1
300	150	2
325	160	3
350	180	4
375	190	5
400	200	6
425	220	7
450	230	8
475	250	9
500	260	

* Celsius (°C) = T (°F)-32] * 5/9

** Fahrenheit (°F) = T (°C) * 9/5 + 32

*** Numbers are rounded to the closest equivalent